Your Child's Best Shot

4TH EDITION

Your Child's Best Shot

A parent's guide to vaccination

Edited by Dorothy L. Moore, MD

Foreword by André Picard

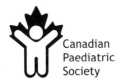

Canadian
Paediatric
Society

Copyright © Canadian Paediatric Society, 2015

All rights reserved. First edition 1997
Fourth edition 2015
ISBN 978-1-926562-03-2 (English paperback)
ISBN 978-1-926562-04-9 (French paperback)

Printed and bound in Canada

Library and Archives Canada Cataloguing in Publication

Your child's best shot (2015)
    Your child's best shot : a parent's guide to vaccination
/ Dorothy L. Moore, editor. – 4th edition.

Includes index.
ISBN 978-1-926562-03-2 (pbk.)

    1. Vaccination of children—Popular works. 2. Vaccines—
Popular works. 3. Communicable diseases—Popular works.
I. Moore, Dorothy L., 1943-, editor II. Canadian Paediatric
Society, issuing body III. Title.

RJ240.Y68 2015   614.4'7083   C2014-904611-1

This book is available in English and French, and may be ordered from the publisher:

Canadian Paediatric Society
2305 St. Laurent Blvd.
Ottawa, Ontario K1G 4J8
Tel. 613-526-9397
Fax 613-526-3332
www.cps.ca, www.caringfokids.cps.ca

Cover and book design: Fairmont House Design
Translation: Dominique Paré (Le bout de la langue)

Please note: The information in this book should be used to support, not to replace, the advice given by a physician, other health professional, or any provincial/territorial health authority. Information is not intended, and should not be used, to contradict specific laws or policies in any jurisdiction. All medical content has been developed by the Canadian Paediatric Society and reviewed by experts.

Website addresses are current as of January 2015

Contents

Tables and text boxes

Tables

Text boxes

Acknowledgements

The Canadian Paediatric Society is profoundly grateful to **Dr. Ronald Gold**, who researched and wrote the first three editions of *Your Child's Best Shot: A Parent's Guide to Vaccination*. His work over more than a decade established the book as a definitive Canadian resource and is both foundation and springboard for the present text.

The 4th edition of *Your Child's Best Shot* was reviewed and revised by members of the **CPS Infectious Diseases and Immunization Committee** for 2013-14.

Special thanks go to the Committee Chair, Joan L. Robinson, MD, Divisional Director, Pediatric Infectious Diseases, University of Alberta, Stollery Children's Hospital, Edmonton, Alta, who provided important input for Part I.

Upton D. Allen, MD, Professor, Pediatrics and Health Policy Management and Evaluation, University of Toronto; Chief, Division of Infectious Diseases, Hospital for Sick Children, Toronto, Ont.

Natalie Bridger, MD, Assistant Professor of Pediatrics, Memorial University; Pediatric Infectious Diseases, Janeway Children's Hospital and Rehabilitation Centre, St. John's, NL; Immunization Monitoring Program, ACTive (IMPACT).

Charles P.S. Hui, MD, Associate Professor, Department of Pediatrics, University of Ottawa; Pediatric infectious disease physician, Children's Hospital of Eastern Ontario, Ottawa, Ont.; Committee to Advise on Tropical Medicine and Travel (CATMAT), Public Health Agency of Canada.

Nicole Le Saux, MD, Associate Professor, Department of Pediatrics, University of Ottawa; Division of Infectious Diseases, CHEO Research Institute, Children's Hospital of Eastern Ontario, Ottawa, Ont.; Immunization Monitoring Program, ACTive (IMPACT)

Noni E. MacDonald, MD, Professor of Pediatrics and Microbiology, Dalhousie University, IWK Health Centre, Halifax, N.S.

Jane C. McDonald, MD, Associate Professor of Pediatrics, Chief, Division of Infectious Diseases and Department of Microbiology, Montreal Children's Hospital, McGill University, Montreal, Que.

Dorothy L. Moore, PhD, MD, Associate Professor of Pediatrics, McGill University; Paediatric infectious disease specialist and associate infection control physician, Montreal Children's Hospital, Montreal, Que.; Immunization Monitoring Program, ACTive (IMPACT).

Heather Onyett, MD, Professor Emeritus, Departments of Pediatrics, Biomedical and Molecular Sciences, and Community Health and Epidemiology, Rehabilitation Therapy, Queen's University, Kingston, Ont.

Portions of this book also benefitted from input from other expert reviewers:

Julie A. Bettinger, PhD, Epidemiologist, Investigator, Vaccine Evaluation Center, CFRI; Associate Professor, Division of Infectious and Immunological Diseases, Department of Pediatrics, University of British Columbia.

Barbara J. Law, MD, Chief – Vaccine Safety, Vaccine and Immunization Program Surveillance Division, Centre for Immunization and Respiratory Infectious Diseases, Public Health Agency of Canada.

Caroline Quach, MD, Associate Professor, Departments of Pediatrics and Epidemiology, Biostatistics and Occupational Health, McGill University; Paediatric infectious disease specialist and infection control physician, Montreal Children's Hospital.

Aline Rinfret, PhD, Chief – Viral Vaccines Division, Biologics and Genetic Therapies Directorate, Health Canada.

David W. Scheifele, OC, MD, Director, Vaccine Evaluation Center, CFRI; Professor, Division of Infectious and Immunological Diseases, Department of Pediatrics, University of British Columbia; Data Centre Chief, IMPACT, Public Health Agency of Canada.

Your Child's Best Shot is available in French under the title ***Les vaccins : Avoir la piqûre pour la santé de votre enfant***. The CPS thanks **Dr. François Boucher**, **Dr. Marc Lebel** and **Dr. Marie-Astrid Lefebvre** for their meticulous review of the French text.

Thanks also to Jennie Strickland, Publications Coordinator, and Elizabeth Moreau, Director, Communications and Public Education with the Canadian Paediatric Society, for their invaluable input and advice, and their limitless patience with the revision of this book.

We thank the **Healthy Generations Foundation** for providing the funds to translate this book into French.

The Canadian Paediatric Society acknowledges, with gratitude, the following **corporate sponsors** for their unrestricted educational grants in support of this publication:
AstraZeneca Canada Inc.
GlaxoSmithKline Inc.
Merck Canada Inc.
Pfizer Canada Inc.

The Canadian Medical Association granted permission to reproduce two copyrighted works adapted from "Reducing the pain of childhood vaccination: An evidence-based clinical practice guideline", *CMAJ* 2010;182(18):E843-55. "Reduce the pain of vaccination in babies: A guide for parents", and "Reduce the pain of vaccination in kids and teens: A guide for parents" are published as an annex to Chapter 4.

Foreword

André Picard

A generation or two ago, vaccination was an easy sell. Infectious disease was omnipresent. So too were the tragic consequences: Large numbers of children sickened, crippled and killed. Parents yearned for protection from common viruses and bacteria that stalked their babies and embraced childhood vaccines as a godsend. So too did hospitals, which were able to shut down their polio and measles wards, and mothball the iron lungs.

The reality is much different today. Once-common childhood illnesses have virtually disappeared from everyday life. The threat posed by pathogens seems more illusory than real. Vaccination feels more like an ordeal than a necessity, anxieties around the side effects of vaccines—real and imagined—seem to have blinded many parents to the benefits, and they are left with nagging doubts about there being too many shots.

It has been said many times, but vaccination is a victim of its own success. Eliminating (and sometimes eradicating) age-old illness is a triumph of science and one of the greatest accomplishments of public health. Mass vaccine campaigns have taken everyday threats—measles, mumps, polio, diphtheria, chickenpox, pertussis, meningitis and more—out of sight and out of mind.

But the flip side is that it is much more difficult to convince parents that these enemies are real, not just historical artifacts, even if they are often invisible.

The challenge for health practitioners today is, more than anything, communicating the continuing value of vaccination. That's not easy, especially given the dramatically different socio-political environment before large-scale immunization campaigns were first introduced.

In the buoyant Baby Boom period, there was unquestioning trust in science and medicine. Even the deaths of several children due to a poisoned batch in the early days of the Salk polio vaccine rollout did not deter enthusiasm. That kind of blind trust no longer exists. Today, many parents fear theoretical harms that may occur from micrograms of preservatives, and they object vociferously to something as mild as a needlestick.

We live in an age of doubt and distrust, especially with "Big Pharma" and "Big Brother" (government), and we no longer show the same deference to "experts" like physicians. We also live in a time when children are safer and healthier than they have ever been and, paradoxically, that has left us fearful and intolerant of any risk, regardless of benefits.

In this environment, it's no surprise that people doubt vaccines.

But we have to remember that vaccine hesitancy has been around, to varying degrees, since the advent of vaccines—since Edward Jenner inserted pus from a cowpox pustule into an incision on a young boy's arm in 1796.

There have always been skeptics and doubters; they are, proportionally, no more numerous today, but they are louder (thanks to amplifying communication technologies like the Internet) and more organized. But there is not, as many believe, a massive anti-vaccination movement.

Virtually every parent wants to protect their child (or children) from harm and they know, intuitively if not scientifically, that vaccination can prevent infections. Sure, there are a few zealots who staunchly oppose vaccination for political or religious reasons, or because they stand to gain financially from promoting so-called "alternative" treatments, but they are a tiny minority.

Only about 2% of parents refuse vaccination outright for their children. But another 10% to 20% of parents delay vaccination or under-vaccinate their children until they are forced to do otherwise (to meet the prerequisites for child care or school admission) because they have doubts or unanswered questions.

This growing demographic of fence-sitters is not ignorant or uneducated—on the contrary. They have legitimate concerns and fears, and having been raised in an era of skepticism, they believe that vaccination is up for negotiation, just like everything else in their lives.

What they don't always have is accurate information, or access to mainstream health professionals who are willing to engage. What they do have is unlimited access to disinformation and a hearty welcome from "alternative" practitioners like homeopaths and some chiropractors, who eschew and belittle vaccination in favour of unproven potions and unscientific promises.

The case of Andrew Wakefield is a classic example. In 1998, he published a research paper in the prestigious medical journal *The Lancet* entitled "Ileal-lymphoid-nodular hyperplasia, non-specific colitis, and pervasive developmental disorder in children". It was a blockbuster. The gastroenterologist examined the cases of 12 children with bowel disease, nine of whom suffered "behavioural abnormalities" shortly after receiving the measles, mumps and rubella vaccine. At a press conference, Dr. Wakefield suggested that the MMR vaccine could trigger autism, particularly in children with intestinal abnormalities. He called for an end to MMR vaccination—the cornerstone of childhood immunization programs—and called for it to be replaced by three separate shots.

The media, and Britain's infamous tabloids in particular, were all over this "perfect storm" of a story, coming as it did when autism rates were soaring, parents were tiring of seeing their children become pincushions for vaccines, and a new communications tool called the Internet was booming.

Scientists around the world diligently tried to reproduce findings from Wakefield's study but never found any evidence of a link between

MMR vaccine and autism. With the passage of time, it became abundantly clear that the research was profoundly flawed, scientifically and ethically. Dr. Wakefield was on the payroll of a law firm that was mounting a class action suit on behalf of "victims" of MMR vaccination, and he had developed a measles vaccine that he was convinced would make him rich.

Though the "research"—fraudulent from beginning to end—was thoroughly discredited, the media coverage (and, truth be told, the rather weak response from public health and the medical establishment) did lasting damage. Fear and doubt are a lot easier to instill than they are to assuage.

But that is the challenge of vaccine providers today: to rebuild trust.

Medical professionals often puzzle at the power and influence of anti-vaccination activists like Jenny McCarthy. What she does is connect on a personal level, speak eloquently to parents about the challenges of parenthood and the tough decisions they have to make. She offers sympathy and support, and a seemingly pain-free alternative.

That is something that few physicians and nurses have the time to do in our increasingly impersonal health system. We tend to treat vaccination as a routine medical act that has to be quickly dispensed with during well-baby visits. That approach disempowers and frightens parents.

With childhood diseases well controlled despite the ever-increasing number of outbreaks, there has to be more basic education. Children need to learn about vaccination in school, not merely lined up for shots occasionally, and serious discussions about vaccination need to occur during the pre-natal period. We need to "prime the pump", if you will.

Vaccines themselves, and the way they are administered, also need to get better. Outbreaks of measles, mumps and pertussis are blamed on anti-vaccinationists, but part of the problem is waning immunity. We do a good job of targeting infants, but the follow-up work—the boosters for teens and young adults—is not done nearly as thoroughly. The pain and discomfort of injected vaccines cannot be dismissed out-of-hand either. When vaccination is a traumatic experience for children (and their parents) it can have a life-long impact on their views.

The good news is that, despite all the challenges, the vast majority of children—90%—*do* get their recommended shots. Vaccines are still saving lives. But faith is wavering, especially in parts of the population that influence public policy.

What the public needs is regular reminders of the benefits of vaccination—"booster shots" if you will—and support for their decisions. Books like *Your Child's Best Shot* are a perfect example of how this can be done. Beyond the printed word, health professionals, and parents themselves, need to engage: to talk openly about the risks and benefits of vaccination and not being vaccinated, to promote and share credible sources of information, and to challenge and denounce the fallacies and myths that are all too common.

Ultimately, parents will make a choice—to have their children vaccinated or not—based on their knowledge and convictions. We have to do everything in our power to ensure that children get their "best shot" at a healthy life.

André Picard is the health columnist at The Globe and Mail, *Canada's national newspaper.*

Introduction

There are many reasons why people will read this book. Some parents are in favour of vaccination but just want to learn more. Some have heard scary stories and want to see what more they can find out. Others are unsure about the need for vaccines in today's world.

There is only one reason this book was written: to inform parents about vaccination with truthful, current, complete and understandable information.

Immunizing children is one of the most important ways to promote their health. Before many of today's vaccines were available, it was not uncommon for children to die or become disabled as a result of infections that are now preventable.

Infections rarely seen in Canada today continue to exist elsewhere in the world. Travellers sometimes bring these germs to Canada, and children may be exposed if they travel to foreign countries. Some germs are still present in older children and adults who don't get seriously ill but may pass their infection on to young children (or the elderly) who can get much sicker. The tetanus germ exists in the soil everywhere, so anyone with an injury is at risk unless they are immunized.

You can't hide from these germs, but you can protect your children through vaccination.

In today's world, there is no shortage of information about vaccines. The difficulty lies in trying to figure out what to believe, especially when every article, website and "official report" has a new angle. The Internet and social media make it easy for people with alarmist views to make unfounded claims, propose unsupported theories or cite false statistics. And it doesn't take long for this information to spread.

In their search for the truth, parents are bound to come across this type of material. But how to distinguish fact from fiction? The purpose of becoming knowledgeable on the subject of vaccines is to help you and your child obtain the best possible health care. To achieve this goal, your decisions must be based on facts—information from reliable authors and sources.

Children are precious. Their health and well-being mean everything. They depend on you to make decisions for them every day, and deciding to vaccinate is a big one. You can't make a decision about vaccination without proper information. You need to know the facts about vaccines *and* disease.

Here, in one book, you'll find important information on childhood infections. It is organized into three main parts, so information is easy to find:

- **Part I** provides general information about vaccination and addresses many issues of concern to parents:
  - Chapter 1 reviews why we vaccinate.
  - Chapters 2 to 6 discuss routine and non-routine vaccinations, the human immune system and how vaccines work, how vaccine safety and effectiveness are monitored, and side effects and common fears about vaccines.

- **Part II** (Chapters 7 to 22) provides complete descriptions of illnesses for which vaccines are routinely given. You'll find everything you need to know about each illness and the vaccine needed to protect against it.
- **Part III** (Chapter 23) has advice on assessing information about vaccines. Several trustworthy websites and other resources are listed here.
- Finally, the **Appendix** gives details about vaccines that may be needed by people who travel to countries where infections are different from those in Canada.

Information in this book is based mainly on the Public Health Agency of Canada's *Canadian Immunization Guide* (the CIG for short). Much of the background information, history and details about diseases are from the third edition of *Your Child's Best Shot*, with updates when appropriate. When information was not available from the CIG, other Public Health Agency of Canada web pages, the 2012 edition of the American Academy of Paediatrics *Red Book*, and the 2013 edition of the classic text *Vaccines* (by Plotkin et al), were used. These resources and others are referenced specifically in Chapter 23.

> **Note**
> The words "vaccination" and "immunization" mean the same thing and are used interchangeably in this book.

This book is written for parents but it does contain scientific material and you may come across some unfamiliar terms. These have been explained using familiar language whenever possible, but you may still have questions about what you read. If you do, please feel free to contact the Canadian Paediatric Society (CPS).

You can connect with the CPS by emailing info@cps.ca, by "liking" us on Facebook, or by following us on Twitter @CanPaedSociety or @CaringforKids (our Twitter account for parents and caregivers).

I

Vaccine basics:
What it's all about

1

Why vaccinate?

Vaccination is one of the most important ways we can protect and promote the health of children. Before vaccines became available, many children died or became disabled as a result of infections that are now preventable.

How serious are the infections discussed in this book?

Very serious! Every disease discussed in this book can cause serious illness, complications and death, even with today's advanced medical care. Many of these diseases have no effective treatment. **Consider these facts about vaccine-preventable diseases in Canada:**

* Healthy children still die from complications of **chickenpox**. Since 2000, there have been 11 reported deaths of children from chickenpox in Canada.

- **Diphtheria** still kills about 1 out of 10 people who get it. In Canada, there are now fewer than 5 cases per year and no deaths since 1992. But diphtheria bacteria have *not* disappeared. Outbreaks still happen, and diphtheria is a significant child health problem in countries with poor vaccine coverage.
- *Haemophilus influenzae* **type b (Hib)** disease is now rare in Canada. In recent years, no more than 16 children under 5 years have had the disease in any given year. But Hib infections, especially meningitis, are dangerous, and fatal cases still happen among unvaccinated children.
- Though on the decline and rarely fatal, **hepatitis A** infection rates are higher among children than other age groups. Hepatitis A is one of the most common infections that travellers pick up when visiting countries where proper sanitation, clean water and safe food are not always available.
- While **hepatitis B** infections have decreased dramatically, they still occur. Children infected with hepatitis B in infancy are usually well for many years, but most develop chronic liver infection, leading to liver failure or cancer later in life.
- **Human papillomavirus (HPV)** is the most common sexually transmitted infection. HPV can cause cancer of the cervix, vulva and vagina in women, cancer of the anus and penis in men, and genital warts.
- **Influenza** comes with every winter and is often a mild infection. But healthy children under 5 years old and older children with a chronic disease, especially a heart or lung disorder, can have severe disease with complications.
- **Measles** outbreaks still happen, with cases reported in five provinces in 2014. Measles can be a serious disease even in healthy, well-nourished children. Today, complications of measles occur in about 10% of cases and death occurs in 1 or 2 of every 1,000 cases. An estimated 140,000 children around the world die from measles each year.
- In recent years, nearly 200 cases of invasive **meningococcal disease** per year were reported in Canada, with death occurring in 7%.
- Large **mumps** outbreaks still happen, especially among young adults. For this group especially, the illness is more severe and complications are more common than in young children. Mumps can cause deafness at any age, and sterility in males.

- **Pertussis** (sometimes called "whooping cough") kills between 1 and 4 infants every year in Canada, and about 1 in 400 survivors suffers permanent brain damage. Older children and adults cope better with this disease than newborns, but they usually suffer several weeks of severe coughing. Reports of outbreaks in pre-adolescents, teenagers and adults have been on the increase since 2010.
- In Canada each year, about 100 children under 5 years old develop serious **pneumococcal disease**. Even with treatment, 10% of children with pneumococcal meningitis will die, and 5% to 10% of survivors have permanent brain damage or deafness.
- The last case of **polio** in Canada was in 1989, but polio still causes disease in three countries, and outbreaks still occur where there is conflict and population displacement. Polio causes permanent paralysis and sometimes, death. Because this infection can be "imported," children in all countries are at risk as long as a single child is infected with polio.
- **Rotavirus** is the main cause of gastroenteritis in children younger than 5 years old, resulting in significant rates of illness and hospitalization, with associated costs.
- A **rubella** outbreak happened in Canada as recently as 2005. Rubella can cause birth defects (heart abnormalities, deafness, blindness, brain damage) or miscarriage if a woman is infected in her first 20 weeks of pregnancy.
- **Tetanus** (sometimes called "lockjaw") still kills 10% to 80% of people who get it. It is rare in Canada—between 1 and 10 cases per year, with only 2 children developing tetanus since 1991. But tetanus spores are everywhere in soil and dust and always will be. In countries that do not vaccinate against tetanus, this disease still kills.

Do breastfeeding and good nutrition prevent these infections?

No! Breastfeeding your baby is not a substitute for vaccination. Breast-feeding provides some protection against many infections because antibodies and immune cells are made in the breasts and passed to an infant in breast milk. Babies who are breastfed generally have lower rates of viral respiratory infections, ear infections and diarrhea. However, the protection provided by breast milk is incomplete, temporary, and can be overcome if a baby is exposed to large amounts of a specific germ.

Good nutrition helps the body's defenses against infection to function normally. Infections are more severe in people with poor nutrition, and malnourished children are much more likely to die of infections such as measles or pertussis than well-nourished children. However, both these infections can also kill or harm healthy, well-nourished children. For example, none of the babies who died of pertussis in the United States in the 1990s were malnourished, and 9 out of 10 children who died in a California outbreak in 2010 were previously healthy.

Do vaccines really work?

Yes! All vaccine-preventable diseases have declined significantly in countries with successful immunization programs. Wherever vaccination rates are high, disease rates are low. Conversely, when vaccination rates decline—whether due to a fear of vaccines or a disruption in health care (e.g., during a war or other disaster)—rates of disease and related deaths always increase.

Vaccines protect **the child** who is immunized, **people close to that child**—such as newborn babies too young to be immunized or others whose immune systems don't work as well—and **the community**, by preventing the spread of disease.

Vaccination can make the world free of some diseases:
• Smallpox was the first disease to disappear because of worldwide vaccination. There have been no cases of smallpox anywhere in the world since 1979. At one time, smallpox vaccine was routine for everyone. Once the disease was gone, this vaccine was no longer necessary.

• Polio has been eliminated from most of the world by vaccination. A global vaccination program is expected to completely eradicate the disease by 2018. If that happens, no one will need polio vaccine in future.

• Measles is next on the list for elimination, but it's proving to be a challenge. The World Health Organization has a goal to eliminate measles from the world by 2020. If vaccine programs around the world are successful, measles vaccine will no longer be needed.

Weren't some of these diseases disappearing long before vaccines became available?

No. Some people think that these infections were disappearing in Canada and other developed countries long before vaccines became available. This is not true.

Until vaccines became available, there was no significant change in the number of cases of these infections.

What had changed before vaccines became available was the *number of deaths* from some of these diseases. Improving socio-economic conditions and better nutrition led to a decline in death rates for some common infections, but not for others. Children still became sick and many had complications. In short, these improvements did not *prevent* disease and deaths still occurred.

If these diseases are now so rare, why do we still need to vaccinate?

These diseases still exist, even if they are rare. Imagine that immunizing a population is like bailing out a boat with a slow leak. When we started bailing (when a vaccine first became available), the boat was full of water (there was a lot of disease). By bailing (vaccinating) the boat became almost dry (the disease became rare). But if we stop bailing, the leak is still there and boat will quickly fill up with water (the disease is still present, and will become common again).

Do I really need to vaccinate my child if so many others are vaccinated?

Yes. Some parents worry unnecessarily about the possible side effects of vaccines. Others don't like to see their child in pain from injections. And widespread vaccination in Canada and other developed countries may give them the mistaken impression that they don't need to vaccinate their own child because so many others are being immunized. This does not work. Here's why:

- Relying on the actions of other parents to protect your unvaccinated child only works if *everyone else* is vaccinated. If many parents take this attitude, fewer children will be immunized and diseases will easily spread.

- While many vaccine-preventable diseases are now uncommon in Canada, they are common in other parts of the world. The speed and ease of air travel, with increasing numbers of people travelling from or immigrating to Canada, pose a real risk of these diseases being brought into Canada, as has happened with polio in the past and with measles in recent years. Any unvaccinated child is at risk when infections are "imported".

- Vaccinating other children does not protect an unvaccinated child from tetanus, for example, which is caused by bacteria in the soil getting into a wound, or from pertussis or chickenpox, which are still infecting older children and adults.

Isn't "natural" better?

Not always. Many providers of homeopathy, naturopathy and other alternative forms of medicine believe that nature's way is best and that "foreign", "unnatural" or "artificial" things like vaccines should be avoided. Some chiropractors also believe this, although the Canadian Chiropractic Association recommends that all children should receive routine immunizations.

The only "infections" that are natural and beneficial involve the many bacteria that live peacefully with us from a few days after we are born. These "normal flora" live on our skin and in our nose, throat, stomach and intestines without making us sick. They are beneficial because they make it harder for other, harmful bacteria to get into our bodies and make certain vitamins for us from the foods we eat.

The bacteria and viruses that make us sick are also part of nature, but like many things in nature, they are harmful, not helpful. Being natural is not always good for human beings. Some of our most potent poisons come from plants and berries.

Vaccines also come from nature. Some are made from live viruses that have undergone changes so that they no longer make us sick. Others are extracted or purified from viruses or bacteria. When injected into the body they stimulate the immune system in a way very similar to the way the infection would, without making us sick.

Still not sure about vaccination?

You are not alone. Many parents have concerns about vaccines. Some are afraid that certain vaccines may harm their child. Others are not sure whether their child really needs all the vaccines being given. Also, there is a tendency for people to fear taking an *action* that they think might cause harm (e.g., vaccination) more than they fear harm that may come from their *inaction* (e.g., not vaccinating).

Parents may also feel understandably confused by conflicting information coming from the Internet or other media sources.

If you have any doubts or concerns, or just feel anxious about vaccinating your child, there are a few steps you can take.

- **Speak with your doctor or a public health nurse as soon as possible.** Tell them why you feel as you do. If they seem unwilling to discuss your concerns, find another doctor or nurse who will. In fact, talking through your concerns even *before* your child is born may help you feel less anxious after your baby arrives.

- **Ask a doctor or nurse what you can do to reduce your child's pain during immunization,** especially when two or three vaccines are being given on the same day. See Chapter 4 of this book for some helpful strategies.

- **Remember that many websites give information that is incorrect or false.** The final chapter in this book offers guidance on how to judge the quality of online (and other) information.

- **If you have decided not to vaccinate, try to keep an open mind.** Parents often feel very differently after their child or a child they know gets a disease that could have been prevented. Sometimes other events (e.g., in the media, discussion with friends, an outbreak of disease) cause parents who have decided not to vaccinate to change their minds. If at any point you want to your discuss your concerns again or reconsider your decisions, don't hesitate to bring this up with a doctor or nurse. They are there to help.

- **Read this book.** It contains a wealth of information from experts you can trust and answers specific questions.

Your Child's Best Shot can also help with perspective. For example, unless you have lived in a country where vaccines are not available for all children, you may never have seen a child who has been damaged by a brain infection from measles or pneumococcus. You may not be aware of what harm such infections can do.

Even if you are already convinced vaccines are dangerous, unnecessary or both, consider reading this book anyway. You may find information here that will change your mind. And even if you don't, you will be more informed than before.

Consequences of deciding not to vaccinate your child

If your child becomes ill and you call or visit a health care provider, be sure to tell them if your child is NOT vaccinated (whether for some or all vaccines). This is to make sure that medical personnel consider the possibility that your child has a vaccine-preventable disease and treat your child appropriately.

If an outbreak—or in some situations a single case—of a vaccine-preventable disease occurs in your community, your child may be asked to stay away from school, child care or other organized activities.

If you know that your child has been exposed to a vaccine-preventable disease, learn what symptoms to watch for and seek immediate medical care if these develop in your child or another family member.

If you travel with your child, learn about possible infection risks at your destination. Certain vaccines may be recommended or required. Also note that children with certain vaccine-preventable diseases, acquired at home or abroad, may be refused permission to travel by public transport (air, train or bus).

2

Routine vaccines: From newborn to grandparent

This chapter outlines vaccines given routinely to healthy children, youth and adults at different periods of life. Detailed descriptions of specific diseases and the vaccines that protect against them are presented in later chapters.

There are a few special circumstances that might affect a child's vaccination schedule.
- Children born outside of Canada may not have received all the vaccines that are routine in this country and might need "catch-up" doses.

- People of any age with certain chronic diseases or conditions may need extra doses of these vaccines, extra vaccines or even different schedules.
- Extra vaccines or doses or different schedules may be needed when the risk of a specific disease is high, for example:
  - When a family travels to certain foreign destinations
  - After close contact with certain infections (such as hepatitis or meningococcal disease)
  - When there is a local outbreak of a vaccine-preventable disease.

More information on special circumstances is in Chapter 3, When extra protection is needed.

Vaccines for infants
(children younger than 1 year old)

Young babies are particularly vulnerable to infection. While they are partially protected by their mother's antibodies, which pass to them in utero shortly before birth and in breast milk after birth, this protection is not effective for all infections. At best, maternal antibody protection is temporary, sometimes lasting for less than 2 months. For other infections, like measles, maternal antibody lasts for up to 12 months.

On the other hand, young infants are often at risk for severe disease from infections that cause a much milder illness in older children or adults.

For these reasons, certain vaccines must be given very early in life, usually starting at 2 months of age, to protect a baby before there's a chance

---

Should I wait until my baby is older to start vaccination?

The purpose of starting at 2 months of age is to protect babies as early in life as possible against diseases to which they are particularly vulnerable. Infants respond well to vaccination at a very young age. Side effects from vaccination *are not* more common in young infants than in older children.

of contact with harmful germs. In special circumstances, some vaccines may be given earlier, even at birth.

The diseases that are most dangerous to young babies are:
- *Haemophilus influenza* type b (Hib), pneumococcus and meningococcus, all of which can cause meningitis, pneumonia and blood infections,
- Rotavirus, a cause of severe diarrhea,
- Pertussis, a cause of severe breathing difficulty,
- Influenza, which causes high fever, febrile seizures and breathing difficulty,
- Diphtheria and tetanus, which are rare but often fatal,
- Polio, a cause of paralysis, eradicated in Canada due to vaccination but which could still be brought into the country at any time,
- Hepatitis B, a liver infection which can eventually cause liver failure or cancer if acquired early in life.

You will find descriptions of these diseases and the vaccines that protect against them in later chapters. For now, here are some things to remember:
- Vaccines against Hib, pertussis, diphtheria, tetanus and polio are combined in one shot. This combination shot is given at 2, 4 and 6 months of age. In some places in Canada, hepatitis B vaccine is added to this combination shot.
- Pneumococcal vaccine is a separate shot given at 2 and 4 months of age.
- Meningococcal vaccine may be given as a separate shot, at 2, 4 and 6 months of age or at 12 months, depending on how much meningococcal disease there is in a specific province, territory or region.
- A separate vaccine against hepatitis B is given in some provinces and territories; others use the combined vaccine referred to above.
- Rotavirus vaccine is given by mouth at 2 and 4 months of age (and sometimes again at 6 months depending on which vaccine brand is used).
- Influenza vaccine does not work in babies under 6 months old, but is given at or after 6 months of age once the influenza season starts, usually in October.

What if my baby is premature?

- Premature infants also respond well to these vaccines and do not have any more side effects than term infants.

- Very premature babies do not get antibodies from their mothers before birth and are especially vulnerable to infections. Immunization should not be delayed and should be given according to the routine schedule, with the exception of hepatitis B vaccine. The response to hepatitis B vaccine may be lower in infants weighing less than 2 kg, and vaccination may be delayed until this weight is reached.

Vaccines for toddlers
(children 1 to 2 years old)

Some vaccines (measles, mumps, rubella and chickenpox) are usually not given before 1 year of age because younger infants do not develop a good immune response after receiving them. For these infections, maternal antibodies usually protect babies for the first 9 to 12 months of life. The measles, mumps and rubella vaccines are only available in a combination shot. Two doses are required, the first when a child is 12 to 15 months old. In some provinces and territories, the second dose is given at 18 months and in others, before starting school at 4 to 6 years of age. Both schedules work well.

Chickenpox vaccine is available in combination with measles, mumps and rubella vaccines as well as on its own. It is given at 12 to 15 months of age. Most provinces and territories provide a second dose at 18 months or before children start school.

Other vaccine doses given to toddlers are "boosters" for vaccines they received as young babies. Boosters are needed because the protection induced by doses given at 2, 4 and 6 months of age does not last very long. Babies receive a pneumococcal booster at one year, plus one combined booster shot for Hib, pertussis, diphtheria, tetanus and polio at 12 to 23 months of age. This booster may also include hepatitis B vaccine in some provinces and territories in Canada.

The meningococcal vaccine may be given for the first time at one year of age. In some provinces and territories, it is given to babies starting at 2 months of age, followed by a booster at 1 year.

Influenza vaccine is given each fall.

Vaccines for preschoolers
(children 4 to 6 years old)

Vaccines given at this age are booster doses for vaccines given earlier. They include:
- Measles, mumps, rubella OR measles, mumps, rubella, chickenpox, unless the child has already received a booster at 18 months. In some jurisdictions, only one dose of chickenpox vaccine is given.
- A combined booster dose of pertussis, tetanus, diphtheria, polio, given as one shot.
- Protection from influenza vaccine is not long-lasting and the vaccine must be given every year. A yearly flu shot is recommended for *all* children. It is provided free of charge for all children under age 2 years in some provinces and territories and all under age 5 years in others, as well as for all children with certain chronic conditions (see Chapter 3, When extra protection is needed). There may be a charge for this vaccine for healthy older children, depending on where you live.

Vaccines for pre-teens and adolescents

- A booster dose of vaccine against pertussis, diphtheria and tetanus is also given to adolescents because protection from the preschool dose has worn off by this age.
- Adolescents are also at risk for serious meningococcal infections, with outbreaks occurring in schools and colleges. A dose of meningococcal vaccine is given, usually at 12 to14 years of age. This vaccine may cover more kinds of meningococcal disease than the one given at 12 months of age.
- A yearly flu shot is recommended.

Some infections are unlikely to occur in younger children but do affect teenagers. These infections may be acquired by sexual activity or risky behaviours, including injection drug use, and are human papillomavirus (HPV), which causes cervical cancer and genital warts, and hepatitis B. Vaccines against both infections are often provided in school programs.

- Hepatitis B vaccine (2 doses, 6 months apart) is given at 8 to 10 years of age to children who were not vaccinated in infancy.
- HPV vaccine is given to girls at 8 to 10 years of age, in 2 or 3 doses, and is provided free of charge. In some jurisdictions, it is also given to boys.

Vaccines for parents

Adults become susceptible to certain infections when immunity from vaccines given earlier in life has waned. Some of these infections, such as diphtheria and tetanus, are severe in all age groups and, although rare, can cause serious damage or death in non-immune adults. Other infections may be mild in adults but can spread to their children.

Infected adults can be a major source of infection for babies.

Some infections, such as pertussis and influenza, can cause a mild illness in adults but pose a serious danger to babies too young to be immunized.

- Adults with pertussis get a persistent, prolonged cough, and are a major cause of spread to babies. Adults should get at least one dose of pertussis vaccine, especially if they are in close contact with young children.
- Adults in close contact with babies and children under 5 years old should get their flu shot each year. The flu shot is recommended for ALL adults.
- Adults need a booster dose of tetanus and diphtheria vaccine every 10 years.

Also, parents who have not received all the recommended childhood and adolescent vaccines should be vaccinated against infections which can cause serious illness in adults, including:

- Polio,
- Measles, mumps, rubella and chickenpox (unless it's known for sure that a parent has had these infections),
- Meningococcal vaccine, if parents are under 25 years old and did not get a booster as an adolescent, especially if they are attending a college or other educational institution,
- Human papillomavirus (HPV), if a parent has not received the vaccine earlier, is under 27 years old OR is at risk of a new exposure.

All routine vaccines can be given safely to breastfeeding mothers.

Vaccines for pregnant women or women planning pregnancy

Some infections have serious consequences for a mother and her newborn (e.g., influenza, hepatitis B, chickenpox), a developing fetus (e.g., rubella), or a newborn (e.g., pertussis).

Some physicians are reluctant to vaccinate pregnant women because they are concerned the developing baby may be harmed. There is *no* evidence that any of the vaccines used routinely today are harmful when given during pregnancy. However, vaccines that contain live viruses (measles, mumps, rubella and chickenpox) are avoided in pregnancy just to be extra cautious.

Planning to get pregnant?

- Make sure to review your vaccine record with a doctor or public health nurse, and if you are missing any vaccines, arrange to get them *before* you become pregnant.
- Ask especially about rubella and chickenpox, infections that can cause serious harm to a developing fetus.
- Also ask about measles and mumps because vaccines for these infections are not given in pregnancy.
- If you don't have a vaccine record, you may need to be vaccinated.

Vaccinating a woman in pregnancy boosts her antibody levels. This boost not only protects her but also means she has more antibodies to pass to her newborn. Because of these higher antibody levels, protection of the newborn lasts longer. Two vaccines are especially beneficial in this way:

- Pertussis vaccine should be given *at least* during the first pregnancy, to women who have not had a dose of pertussis vaccine as an adult. This booster also protects the pregnant woman from the stressful chronic cough that pertussis causes in adults.
- Influenza vaccine protects the newborn while protecting the mother against severe influenza. The vaccine should be given during each pregnancy.

Vaccines for grandparents

Grandparents play an important role in a child's life. Besides receiving vaccines to protect their own health, they need vaccines to protect against infections that could pass easily to a grandchild:

- Influenza can cause severe infection in older adults *and* in the young babies they are in contact with or caring for. All grandparents, regardless of age, need yearly flu vaccine if they are in contact with children under 5 years old. People 65 years of age and over and younger adults with selected chronic conditions should also get the flu shot each year. It is provided free of charge for these groups.
- Grandparents need a booster dose of pertussis vaccine if they have not received one as an adult.
- Diphtheria and tetanus are rare but severe diseases more likely to occur in the elderly, who have either lost immunity over time or never been immunized. Everyone who has not received a dose of diphtheria or tetanus vaccine in the past 10 years should get one. This shot is usually given in combination with pertussis.
- Pneumococcus causes severe pneumonia and death in the elderly. A dose of pneumococcal vaccine is recommended for all adults at age 65.
- Shingles (or zoster) is a painful condition caused by reactivation of the chickenpox virus in older adults. Adults with shingles can infect non-immune children, who then develop chickenpox. The shingles

vaccine is recommended for adults 60 years of age and over (the age group most likely to get shingles) but can be given earlier, starting at age 50. People usually have to pay for shingles vaccine but the cost is covered by some insurance policies. Ask your health care provider or pharmacist for details.

3

When extra protection is needed

In some situations, the protection provided by routine vaccines described in Chapter 2 is not enough, either because children have underlying medical conditions or because they are at risk of exposure to certain infections during an outbreak or while travelling. These situations are described in this chapter, along with how optimal protection can be achieved.

Chronic medical conditions

Some children with chronic conditions, whether present from birth or developing later on, need extra protection against infection. Which vaccines they need depends on the medical condition. Certain infections can cause children with a chronic condition to be more severely ill than other children, or to have a more serious disease at an older age than other children. Your child's physician or a public health nurse may have already discussed these risks with you.

Table 3.1 (at the end of this section) has "at-a-glance" guidance for protecting people with chronic conditions, while the condition-specific sections below provide some explanation and details.

It is important for children and adolescents who have a chronic condition and a *normal immune system* to be fully immunized with both live and inactivated vaccines and in accordance with routine immunization schedules. In some cases, however, additional vaccines, additional doses or higher dosages are needed to protect children with certain conditions. Vaccination is best done early on, when their immune responses are more likely to resemble those in children of a similar age with no chronic condition. If certain chronic conditions progress, sometimes vaccines don't work as well.

Some children have more than one of the conditions discussed below. For information on vaccinating individuals with conditions or undergoing treatments that suppress the immune system, see "Immunocompromising conditions" later in this chapter.

Do you live with someone who has a chronic medical condition?

To prevent someone in your home from catching an infection that they might then pass on to a more vulnerable person, *all* family members and household contacts should get *all* the routine immunizations *and* the yearly influenza vaccine (flu shot).

Chronic lung disease

Children and adolescents with lung disease may become very ill if they develop lung infections (pneumonia), often caused by pneumococci or influenza. People with diseases such as bronchopulmonary dysplasia, severe asthma, cystic fibrosis or chronic obstructive pulmonary disease are at higher risk of complications from influenza and pneumococcal infections.

- They should get influenza vaccine (the flu shot) each fall.
- All children and adolescents (up to 18 years of age) should get the conjugate pneumococcal vaccine (which covers 13 types of pneumococci) unless they received it in early childhood. Normally, this vaccine is only given to healthy children under 5 years old.
- All children older than 2 years of age should also get the polysaccharide vaccine (which covers 23 types of pneumococci). The polysaccharide vaccine is also given to adults with chronic lung disease.

People with cystic fibrosis are also at risk of complications from chickenpox. They should get the chickenpox (varicella) vaccine if they have not had the vaccine (or the disease) in the past.

Chronic heart disease

Children and adolescents with heart disease, caused either by an abnormality present at birth or a disease later in life, are at risk for cardiac failure if they develop infections, especially pneumonia. Individuals with a cardiac disorder should get:
- Influenza vaccine (the flu shot) every year.
- Conjugate and polysaccharide pneumococcal vaccines, as outlined above for people with chronic lung disease.

Chronic kidney disease

Infections can have serious effects in children and adolescents with severe kidney disease or who require dialysis. In one form of kidney disease called "nephrotic syndrome", antibodies and other proteins are rapidly lost. People who have kidney failure are at higher risk for complications from influenza, pneumococcal disease and hepatitis B.

Individuals with chronic kidney disease should get:
- Influenza vaccine (the flu shot) every year.

- Conjugate and polysaccharide pneumococcal vaccines, as outlined above for people with chronic lung disease.
- Hepatitis B vaccine *as early as possible*, if they did not receive this vaccine in infancy. The immune response to hepatitis B vaccine in people with kidney failure is not as good as in others, so higher than usual doses are needed to stimulate their immune response.

Spleen problems, chronic anemia and bleeding disorders

The spleen is an organ in the abdomen that helps the body eliminate some types of bacteria, especially Hib, pneumococci and meningococci. Some children are born without a spleen. Others have had their spleen removed surgically because of a traumatic injury or disease. The spleen may also be damaged and unable to function normally in people who have a blood disorder where red blood cells are abnormal (e.g., sickle cell anemia, thalassemia and some other chronic anemias).

People who don't have a normal spleen are at higher risk for overwhelming bacterial infection, which can be rapidly fatal. The risk is highest in young children but it lasts life-long.
- Hib vaccine is given to healthy children only up to 5 years old. But individuals with a defective spleen, regardless of age, should receive a Hib booster at or after age 5, or a single dose if they are 5 years of age or older and received no Hib vaccine previously.
- They should also get conjugate pneumococcal vaccine *regardless of age* and polysaccharide pneumococcal vaccine at age 2 years or older.
- Healthy children routinely receive only group C meningococcal vaccine as infants, and healthy adolescents get type C or quadrivalent (A-C-Y-W135) meningococcal vaccine depending on the types of meningococci present in the region where they live. People whose spleen isn't working normally should be given the quadrivalent meningococal vaccine *as soon as the problem is recognized*. This vaccine can be given safely to children as young as 2 months old.

- Having influenza makes people more likely to get the bacterial infections described above. Anyone with a spleen problem should receive influenza vaccine (the flu shot) every year.
- Chickenpox may be complicated by bacterial infections. People who have not been immunized and have not had chickenpox should get the chickenpox (varicella) vaccine.
- Some people with chronic anemia or bleeding disorders need frequent transfusions of blood or blood products. They should get hepatitis A and hepatitis B vaccines.

If surgery to remove the spleen is planned (i.e., not an emergency surgery), all required vaccines should be given *at least* 2 weeks before the operation.

In the case of an emergency spleen removal, vaccines are best given 2 weeks *after* the surgery. It is important not to forget about immunization when the child or adolescent is sent home from hospital to recuperate during the two-week period after surgery.

Chronic liver disease

Liver cells, which play an important role in removing bacteria from the bloodsteam, may not work well in people with chronic liver disease, leaving these individuals at high risk for pneumococcal infections. Getting hepatitis A or B after having chronic liver disease from another cause can lead to rapid liver failure. People with chronic liver disease should get:
- Influenza vaccine (the flu shot) every year.
- Conjugate and polysaccharide pneumococcal vaccines, as outlined above for people with chronic lung disease.
- Hepatitis A and hepatitis B vaccines.

All these vaccines should be given *as early as possible* because they may not work as well when someone has advanced liver disease.

Neurologic disorders

In addition to routine immunizations:
- Children and adolescents with a chronic neurologic disorder should get the flu shot each year.

- People of any age who have a condition that makes it difficult to control respiratory secretions or that causes aspiration (inhaling material into the lungs) should receive yearly influenza vaccine, as well as conjugate and polysaccharide pneumococcal vaccines, as outlined above for people with chronic lung disease.
- Individuals with a chronic cerebrospinal fluid (CSF) leak should receive conjugate and polysaccharide pneumococcal vaccines, as outlined above for people with chronic lung disease.

Diabetes

People with diabetes mellitus (type 1 or 2) are at risk for complications from influenza and pneumococcal infections. Infections also make managing blood sugar much more difficult. Children and adolescents living with diabetes should get:

- Influenza vaccine (the flu shot) every year.
- Conjugate and polysaccharide pneumococcal vaccines, as outlined above for people with chronic lung disease.

Chronic inflammatory diseases

Chronic inflammatory diseases include some types of arthritis and inflammatory bowel disease, among others. Infections are a common cause of illness and hospitalization for people living with these disorders. Respiratory tract infections, including influenza and pneumococcus, are the most common. People *not* receiving treatment that suppresses the immune system should be given all routine vaccines as early as possible in the course of their disease. That's because their immune response won't be as strong later on if they need immunosuppressive treatment. In addition to all routine vaccines, they should get:

- Influenza vaccine (the flu shot) every year.
- Conjugate and polysaccharide pneumococcal vaccines, as outlined above for people with chronic lung disease.
- Hepatitis B vaccine.
- Chickenpox (varicella) vaccine, if they are not already immune.

People being treated with immunosuppressive therapy should not receive live vaccines. Inactivated vaccines are safe but they may not work as well if given before treatment is started. For more information, see "Immunocompromising conditions" below.

Salicylate therapy

Long-term salicylate treatment with aspirin or related drugs is sometimes used to control chronic inflammatory disease and other conditions. A condition called Reye's syndrome, which causes liver failure and brain damage, has been associated with influenza and chickenpox *infections* (not vaccines) in young people who were taking salicylates. While Reye's syndrome has *never* been reported after a child or teen has received live influenza or chickenpox vaccines, there is a theoretical concern that this might happen.

For children and adolescents taking salicylates:
• Inactivated influenza vaccine should be used.
• Unfortunately, there is no alternative to the live vaccine for chickenpox. The vaccine may be considered for young people who are likely to be exposed to chickenpox, as there is a known risk of Reye's syndrome with the disease.

Cancer

People with cancer are likely to have more severe infections. Many types of cancer, especially those common in children, affect the immune system. Cancer treatments also have very serious effects on the immune system. For discussion of vaccination and cancer, see "Immunocompromising conditions" below.

Cochlear implants

People who are deaf and have (or will be receiving) a cochlear implant—a device implanted near the ear to help restore hearing—are more likely to get pneumococcal or Hib meningitis. In addition to *all* routine vaccines, they should get:
• Both the conjugate and polysaccharide pneumococcal vaccines, as outlined above for people with chronic lung disease.
• A dose of Hib vaccine at or after 5 years of age, regardless of age or the number of previous doses.

Table 3.1
Vaccines recommended for children and adolescents with selected chronic medical conditions

Condition	Influenza every year	Pneumococcus		Hib booster if ≥5 yrs	Meningococcus quadrivalent conjugate vaccine	Chickenpox if not immune	HBV	HAV
		Conjugate 13 serotypes	Polysaccharide 23 serotypes if age >2 yrs					
Chronic lung disease	✔	✔ if age <18 yrs	✔					
Cystic fibrosis	✔	✔ if age <18 yrs	✔			✔		
Chronic heart disease	✔	✔ if age <18 yrs	✔					
Chronic kidney disease	✔	✔ if age <18 yrs	✔				✔ higher dose	
Spleen problems, chronic anemia, bleeding disorder	✔	✔ any age	✔	✔	✔	✔		
Frequent transfusions							✔	✔
Chronic liver disease	✔	✔ if age <18 yrs	✔				✔	✔
Neurologic disorder*	✔	✔ if age <18 yrs	✔					
Diabetes (type 1 or 2)	✔	✔ if age <18 yrs	✔					
Chronic salicylate therapy	✔							
Chronic inflammatory disease	✔	✔ if age <18 yrs	✔			✔	✔	
Cochlear implant	✔	✔ if age <18 yrs	✔	✔				

* For specific conditions

Immunocompromising conditions

People who have an immune system that does not work well are considered to be "immunocompromised". They may have been born with an immune disorder—known as congenital immunodeficiency—or they may have an acquired immunodeficiency, caused by:

- an illness they got later on, or
- a treatment that is immunosuppressive, such as chemotherapy.

Immunocompromised people are at higher risk for severe illness from many vaccine-preventable infections. This section helps to explain why vaccines are given differently to children or adolescents whose immune systems do not work well.

The degree of immunocompromise can vary depending on a person's condition and may change over time. Your doctor will discuss your child's particular issues with you.

> **First, do no harm**
> The goal when vaccinating an immunocompromised person is to provide the maximum possible protection without causing harm.

The following general principles apply when vaccinating a child or adolescent whose immune system isn't working well:

- Inactivated vaccines are safe to give. They do not contain live germs that could multiply and cause disease. However, immune response to these vaccines may be weaker than that in a healthy child, so more doses or larger doses of a vaccine may be needed to maximize protection.
- Live vaccines can sometimes cause disease in immunocompromised individuals, if the vaccine virus multiplies too extensively and especially if their condition is severe. Live vaccines are usually not given, with a few exceptions.
- An immunocompromised child may need vaccines that are not routinely given to all children or are not routinely given after a certain age.

- Length of immunity after a vaccine is given may be shorter than normal, making extra booster doses necesssary.
- The timing of vaccination depends on when a person's best response can be expected. This may mean giving vaccines later than usual if the immune function is expected to improve, or earlier than usual if:
  - the immune function is likely to weaken further, or
  - before starting immunosuppressive therapy.
- Extra protection may be needed if, for example, an immuno-compromised child is exposed to chickenpox at school or in day care. In this case, an injection of immune globulin (a blood product containing a high concentration of chickenpox antibodies) would be given.
- Extra vaccines may be required for foreign travel because immuno-compromised people are at higher risk of infection in parts of the world where infections differ from those in Canada (see "Vaccines for travellers", below, and the Appendix to this book).

Do you live with someone who is immunocompromised?

All household and other close contacts of an immunocompromised person should receive *all* routine immunizations, on time, to prevent them from infecting a more vulnerable family member or friend. They should also get:
- Influenza vaccine (the flu shot) every year.
- Hepatitis B vaccine, if not already given.

Congenital immunodeficiency

Congenital immunodeficiencies include problems with antibodies or complement (proteins that help destroy some types of bacteria), or with lymphocytes (white blood cells crucial to the immune system), and conditions where neither antibodies nor lymphocytes work well. Children born with an immunodeficiency are very susceptible to pneumococcal, Hib and meningococcal infections. Children born with lymphocyte defects are also susceptible to all viruses and many bacteria.
- Children with antibody defects may be protected from many infections by regular infusions of immune globulin.

- Children with lymphocyte defects and some types of antibody deficiency are not given live vaccines. Inactivated vaccines are safe but may not work.
- Children with other types of antibody deficiency and normal lymphocyte responses may get live and inactivated vaccines, although they may not work as well as in someone with normal immune function. If children have some (though reduced) antibody function, vaccination is recommended to raise antibody levels.

  In addition to all routine inactivated vaccines, these individuals should get:
  - Conjugate pneumococcal, Hib and hepatitis B vaccines, regardless of age.
  - Inactivated influenza vaccine yearly.
  - Polysaccharide pneumococcal vaccine, if they are 2 years of age and older.
  - Quadrivalent conjugate meningococcal (A-C-Y-W135) vaccine (rather than meningococcal C vaccine).
- People with an isolated complement deficiency can get *all* live and inactivated vaccines. They should also get the quadrivalent conjugate meningococcal vaccine (rather than meningococcal C vaccine).
- People with isolated phagocyte or neutrophil disorders but normal lymphocyte responses may receive all inactivated vaccines and live viral vaccines but not live bacterial vaccines, which are sometimes used for foreign travel.

Acquired immunodeficiency

Acquired immunodeficiencies are caused by a disease or treatment that affects the immune system, such as cancer, HIV infection, a stem cell or organ transplant, chemotherapy, or other immunosuppressive treatments.

Cancer patients are immunocompromised by disease or by chemotherapy. Inactivated vaccines can be given according to routine schedules, but they may not work as well. As well, these patients should receive:
- Pneumococcal conjugate, Hib and hepatitis B vaccines, regardless of age.

- Inactivated influenza vaccine, yearly.
- Polysaccaharide pneumococcal vaccine, if they are 2 years of age and older.

Live vaccines are generally *not* given, with a few exceptions:
- Children with acute lymphocytic leukemia may be vaccinated with measles, mumps, rubella and chickenpox (varicella) vaccines if their disease has been in remission for at least a year and certain other criteria are met.
- People with cancer in remission and off chemotherapy for at least 3 months can usually be given live vaccines.

Hematopoietic stem cell transplantation (HSCT) of blood or bone marrow stem cells is often used to treat cancer or a congenital immunodeficiency. Treatment required before transplant destroys a person's immune system and a new immune system needs to develop after the transplant. Vaccination must then start over again. The immune system starts to function some months after transplantation.
- Inactivated vaccines, including influenza vaccine, are usually started 6 to 12 months after transplant surgery.
- Live vaccines are usually started at 24 months.
- All HSCT recipients are at risk for infections that usually affect young children and should receive conjugate and polysaccharide pneumococcal, Hib and meningococcal vaccines, regardless of age.

Solid organ transplant recipients are at risk for severe illness or death due to influenza, invasive pneumococcal disease, Hib disease and complications of chickenpox. Ideally, any child waiting for a new kidney, lung, liver or heart should be immunized before the transplantation and as early as possible. Vaccine response is lower as an organ fails, so this may be the best chance to protect the child.

Usually, immune suppression is greatest in the first 3 to 6 months after a transplant, but significant immune suppression persists for life. If vaccines are still missing, inactivated vaccines can usually be started at

3 to 6 months after a transplant, once immunosuppression has been stabilized. Live vaccines are not given after organ transplant, with a very few exceptions.

In addition to all routine vaccines, organ transplant recipients should receive:
• Hib and conjugate pneumococcal vaccines, regardless of age.
• Polysaccharide pneumococcal vaccine, if 2 years of age or older.
• Inactivated influenza vaccine, yearly.
• Hepatitis B vaccine, if not already received.
• Hepatitis A vaccine for liver transplant cases.

> **Vaccines work better if they are given before transplantation**
>
> The medications that need to be taken for life after an organ transplant, to prevent rejection, are immunosuppressive. For optimal protection, inactivated vaccines should be given *at least* 2 weeks before, and live vaccines *at least* 4 weeks before, transplantation.

HIV infection causes widely varying degrees of immune suppression, which can be measured using blood tests.

Whenever possible, vaccines are given early in the course of infection if immune function is good. If not so good, vaccines are given after immune function has been restored by antiretroviral HIV treatment. Inactivated vaccines can be given at any time but they may not work well if immune function is weak. Routine live vaccines are not given if immune function remains poor. All other routine vaccines should be given, as well as:
• A yearly flu shot (live or inactivated, depending on an individual's immune function).
• Conjugate and polysaccharide pneumococcal vaccines.
• Hib vaccine.
• Quadrivalent conjugate meningococcal vaccine, in some cases.

Immunosuppressive treatments include cancer chemotherapy, long-term high-dose steroids given by mouth, and immunosuppressive drugs for chronic inflammatory disorders.

People undergoing immunosuppressive therapy are at high risk of invasive pneumococcal disease and influenza-related complications.

Vaccine records should be reviewed for anyone with a disease that might later require immunosuppressive treatment. In addition to routine vaccines, these individuals should receive:
• Conjugate and polysaccharide pneumococcal vaccines.
• Inactivated influenza vaccine, yearly.
• Hib vaccine in some circumstances.

Ideally, all appropriate vaccines or boosters should be given before starting treatment. Inactivated vaccines should be given *at least* 14 days before, and live vaccines *at least* 4 weeks before, treatment starts.

If these vaccines cannot be given before treatment is started, they should be delayed until *at least* 3 months after treatment has finished (4 weeks if the treatment is high-dose steroids only). The interval between stopping treatment and giving vaccines will vary with the type of treatment and the underlying disease.

If treatment includes injected immunosuppressive monoclonal antibodies (e.g., rituximab, infliximab, adalimumab), immunosuppression can last for many months after the last injection.

If immunosuppressive therapy cannot be stopped, inactivated vaccines may be given when the person is on their lowest dose of the treatment. An exception would be when a vaccine is urgently needed because of exposure to an infection. Live vaccines are generally not given.

Exposures and outbreaks

When exposures or outbreaks occur, health professionals may need to take urgent steps to prevent the infection from spreading.

An **exposure** means that someone has been in close contact with a specific infection, usually from a family member but sometimes from a person in child care or at school.

Here are some examples of exposures and how they are managed:
- An unimmunized child in contact with someone with chickenpox, measles, pertussis, hepatitis A or hepatitis B may need to get the vaccine against that infection.
- If in contact with someone with meningococcus, a booster dose may be needed, even if the exposed child has already been vaccinated.
- If someone is injured, especially if the wound is contaminated with dust or soil, a tetanus vaccine booster may be needed.

In cases where vaccine can't be given or may not work, antibodies (immune globulin) are given by injection.
- Immune globulin may be needed after contact with chickenpox, hepatitis A or measles.
- For hepatitis B and tetanus, both vaccine *and* immune globulin may be needed.

For some infections (e.g., meningococcus), antibiotics are required for close contacts.

For more information, see chapters on specific infections and "Passive immunity" in Chapter 4.

An **outbreak** means that there is an unusually high number of cases of a specific infection in a community. Extra booster doses of a vaccine may be given or vaccines that are not routine may be used to control an outbreak. For example:
- In mumps outbreaks, vaccine has been given to all people in the community who had received only one dose in the past.
- Meningococcal vaccines have been used in large immunization campaigns to control outbreaks in several provinces or territories. A new meningococcal group B vaccine was used to control a regional outbreak in Quebec in 2014.

- In the 2009 worldwide influenza outbreak (pandemic), a new pandemic influenza vaccine was used throughout Canada.

For more information, see chapters on specific infections.

Vaccines for foreign travel

Parents planning foreign travel with their children, especially to places where infection risks are high or infections are different from those in Canada (e.g., Africa and some parts of Asia and South America), should discuss their plans with a physician. Ideally, this talk should happen at least 6 weeks before leaving. But even if families leave on short notice, a pre-travel consultation is strongly recommended.

This section offers an overview of vaccination for travellers. You may also want to learn about protecting your family against insect bites, malaria, injuries, heat stroke, altitude sickness and food- or water-borne illnesses. Consider visiting a travel health clinic or talking to a specialist in travel medicine. You can also find information online, such as at: http://travel. gc.ca/travelling/health-safety/children.

For routine vaccines, schedules may change

Each family member should already have received all the routine vaccines appropriate for their age. If any vaccines or doses are missing, these should be given before travelling.

Many diseases now rare in Canada because of vaccines (such as measles and diphtheria) are still common in other countries. Children who travel are likely to be exposed to these infections.

Some vaccines may need to be given earlier than usual. For example, measles vaccine is given to children as young as 6 months old when they are travelling to places where measles is common. Other vaccines may be given on an accelerated (speeded-up) schedule, starting at 6 weeks of age.

In Canada, all children are given hepatitis B vaccine, but the age at which they get it varies. Hepatitis B vaccine is recommended for all children who are not yet immunized but who are going to live in an area where this disease is common: the Far East, the Middle East, Africa, South America, and parts of Eastern Europe and Central Asia. Short-term travellers who will have close contact with family or other residents and may have accidental exposure to their blood, or who may have sexual contact, should also receive hepatitis B vaccine. For more information on hepatitis B virus and vaccine, see Chapter 11.

Travel vaccines may be needed

Other vaccines are recommended for travellers to parts of the world where certain infections are much more common than in Canada.

For advice about which travel vaccines are needed for a specific country and whether your child should get them, consult with your doctor or local public health department. Reliable, current information is also available from the Public Health Agency of Canada (visit www.phac-aspc.gc.ca/ tmp-pmv/and www.phac-aspc.gc.ca/publicat/cig-gci/p03-10-eng.php) or the U.S. Centers for Disease Control and Prevention (visit wwwnc. cdc.gov/travel).

Some travel-related infections, such as **hepatitis A, meningococcus** and **typhoid**, are more likely to occur in child travellers than in adults.

Yellow fever vaccine is required for entry into certain countries.

Additional travel vaccines are sometimes needed, depending on destination, how long a traveller will be away (especially if moving to another country), living conditions, what a traveller will be doing (e.g., hiking or working), and the chance of exposure to biting insects or to animals. Such vaccines include **Japanese encephalitis vaccine, tick-borne encephalitis vaccine, cholera and travellers' diarrhea vaccine, rabies vaccine**, and **the tuberculosis vaccine Bacille Calmette-Guérin (BCG)**.

Children living with a chronic disease or who are immunocompromised may require extra vaccines for travel.

Brief descriptions of each disease (except for hepatitis A and meningo-coccal disease, which are described in Chapters 10 and 15) are provided in the Appendix to this book, along with information about the vaccine to prevent it, recommendations on who should receive the vaccine and, in some cases, who should not.

4

The ABCs of vaccines

Most parents wonder how a needle filled with fluid keeps their child safe from disease. This chapter will help you understand just that.

The goal of a vaccine is to make a person immune to a germ, which means if they get the germ, it will not make them sick. To understand how this is possible, you first have to know how the immune system works.

How vaccines work

The immune system

The immune system helps protect the body against infection. Its job is to identify and remove foreign substances (such as germs) from the body. The germs causing the diseases described in this book are either bacteria or viruses.

Germs

Bacteria are microscopic organisms—they are too tiny to be seen with our eyes alone. They are "complete" in that they are able to live on their own as long as they have a food supply to nourish them.

Viruses, on the other hand, are "incomplete" organisms, meaning they cannot live on their own. To grow and reproduce, the virus must get inside a cell. Once inside, the virus takes over the function of the cell and uses it to make new virus particles.

Bacteria and viruses have unique proteins and polysaccharides (complex sugars) on their surfaces called **antigens**. These are very different from human proteins and sugars:
- Some surface antigens allow the germ to stick to human cells. This is the first step of infection.
- Other antigens protect the germ against the body's defences. Our immune system targets these antigens.

The body's defences
Initial response

The immune system's initial response to infecting germs is to destroy them and help the body recover from infection. It does this by producing antibodies (a type of protein), and special white blood cells called lymphocytes.

Antibodies attach to the surface of the germ and kill it, either by damaging it directly or by allowing other white blood cells to kill the germ. The immune system can also make specific antibodies that attach to toxins (poisons) produced by germs. Antibodies block the action of the toxin and make it easier for the body to get rid of it.

Lymphocytes are white blood cells that act as the "backbone" of the immune system. Some, called B-lymphocytes or B-cells, make antibodies; others, called T-lymphocytes or T-cells, have a number of different jobs. For example, they help the immune system to identify the presence of bacteria and viruses. They also stimulate the B-cells to grow, multiply and produce more antibodies. Other T-cells recognize cells that are infected with a germ, and kill both the infected cell and the germ.

Initial immunity takes time

Unfortunately, it takes time for the body to develop antibodies and the right kind of lymphocytes. Sometimes a bad infection kills the person or causes severe damage before the immune response can kick in.

Long-term response: Immune memory

A second function of the immune system is to establish immune memory.

Memory cells are another important group of lymphocytes. They live a very long time, sometimes for life. Memory cells allow the immune system to recognize a germ it has seen before—even many years ago—so that it can respond immediately, producing antibodies and lymphocytes to attack germs quickly and kill them before they cause damage. The memory cells create long-lasting immunity to an infection, which is called "immune memory". When immune memory has been established, a person is "immune" to that disease.

It is important to understand that immune memory is very specific. Each germ triggers a unique response in the immune system. A separate, distinct set of antibodies, T-cells, B-cells and memory cells are programmed to detect and react to one, and only one, type of germ.

Immunity is infection-specific

Becoming immune to one infection does not create immunity to other infections. Antibodies and lymphocytes made in response to measles infection or measles vaccine react only to measles virus and will not fight off chickenpox.

Two ways to immunity

There are two ways to achieve immunity: by natural infection and by vaccine. Now that you know how the immune system works, you may wonder whether there is a difference in the immunity achieved by vaccine as opposed to infection. To illustrate how natural infections and vaccines produce a very similar end result—long-term immunity—let's use measles as an example.

Natural infection. The first time someone is exposed to the natural form of the measles virus, the virus infects many cells and causes illness in the person before the immune response can develop. Infection from measles can do a lot of damage. In severe cases, the infection spreads so rapidly that the person dies before immunity can be established. Once a person has had measles and survived, long-term immunity is established. Immunity after measles infection lasts a very long time, usually for life.

The terms **vaccination** and **immunization** mean the same thing and are used interchangeably in this book. With immunization, a person's immune system is deliberately exposed to a vaccine containing inactive or weakened germs or parts of germs. They cause the immune system to respond just as it would to the actual infection, creating long-term immunity without a person's having to get the disease. Vaccines stimulate antibodies and lymphocytes so that they are present in the body *before* exposure to an infection occurs. Following vaccination, the immune system responds as if natural infection has already occurred.

For example, after the measles vaccine is injected into a person, it stimulates antibodies and lymphocytes and creates long-term immunity. The person may have a little redness and swelling at the injection site, and possibly a mild fever and rash. Measles vaccine establishes immunity to the illness that usually lasts for life, without causing measles.

Is immunity from natural infection the same as immunity from vaccine?

Yes. Although there are two ways of achieving immunity, the end result is the same. A person will be immune to measles after either natural infection with measles virus or after receiving the measles vaccine. If that person is exposed to the measles virus again, the immune system will respond so quickly that the virus is destroyed before it can cause infection.

The main difference between natural infection and vaccination is that the person who receives the vaccine does not endure the illness or its complications, which can be life-threatening.

Opponents of vaccination often claim that natural immunity from an infection is better than immunity from a vaccine. But in fact, immunity after most vaccines is just as effective as that induced by the disease.

Every infection described in this book has great potential to cause harm. The truth is that the proven risks of damage and death caused by the disease itself are *far worse* than the so-called "benefits" of obtaining immunity through disease.

There may be a difference in the *amount* of antibody made after infection compared with after vaccine, but the same *kinds* of antibodies and immune cells are made. Also, because some young children may not make enough antibodies after their first dose of measles vaccine, a second dose is given to ensure life-long immunity to measles.

Do all vaccines produce the same level of immunity as in this measles example?

Not exactly. While measles infection and measles vaccine produce similar immunity, some vaccines are not as effective as measles vaccine in preventing infection. Rather, they modify the illness so that if infection develops after vaccine, it is very much milder and less likely to cause harm than if the person was not vaccinated.

Does immunity wear off over time?

Sometimes. Antibody levels in the blood decline over time after both natural infection and vaccination. But even when antibodies disappear, immune memory lasts. Many vaccines produce immune memory that lasts a very long time, often for life.

Sometimes, booster doses are necessary. Certain vaccines, such as diphtheria and tetanus toxoid vaccine, must be repeated to maintain protection against disease. These repeated doses are called "boosters". Boosters create antibody and immune lymphocytes quickly and enhance immune memory.

Tetanus and diphtheria are different from most other infections described in this book in the way they cause disease. Both cause illness by producing a toxin (or poison). These toxins are so potent that disease can occur before the immune system has time to make antibodies. Protection against these diseases requires the actual presence of antibodies in the blood at the time a person is exposed to the toxin. Boosters are needed every 10 years to keep antibody levels high enough to protect against diphtheria and tetanus.

> ### Some vaccines are much better than natural infection at stimulating immunity
>
> The toxin (poison) produced by tetanus germs is so powerful that only a tiny amount causes disease, an amount so small that it cannot stimulate an immune response. Therefore, having tetanus does not induce immunity.
>
> This sometimes happens with diphtheria as well.

Won't adults be at risk of catching these infections if immunity wears off?

Perhaps. But this sometimes happens after natural infection as well as after vaccines.

Booster doses of some vaccines, especially tetanus and diphtheria, are already recommended for adults. Other infections such as measles, mumps, rubella and chickenpox are more severe in adults than in children, and adults may be at risk if immunity from their childhood vaccines wears off.

While immune memory from measles and rubella vaccines can last a lifetime, the situation is less clear for mumps and chickenpox. An outbreak of mumps among college students in the United States in 2006 seemed to result from waning vaccine immunity over time. And some children vaccinated against chickenpox as infants have developed mild chickenpox several years later.

Medical surveillance systems in Canada and the United States watch out for cases of vaccine-preventable disease in all age groups. If infections begin to show up in adults who were vaccinated as children, vaccination programs will be adjusted to provide booster doses for adults.

Can vaccines "wear out" the immune system?

No! The human immune system has a truly awesome capacity to recognize the different proteins and polysaccharides known as antigens. It can respond to intense and repeated stimulation each and every day. The food we eat, the air we breathe and the water we drink are filled with antigens that our immune system recognizes as familiar or foreign. Its job is to respond appropriately by helping the body get rid of any foreign substances.

Scientists estimate that human infants can respond to about 10,000 different antigens at any one time. A dose of vaccine is unlikely to challenge the immune system any differently from other foreign antigens in the daily load entering the body, even in a 2-month-old baby.

The vaccines used today are also much more highly purified than in the past, so they have fewer antigens. Even though infants and children receive more vaccines now than 30 years ago, the total numbers of antigens the immune system must deal with is much lower than it used to be.

Frequent vaccination has been closely studied

A group of employees working in a United States army laboratory were examined for effects of repeated immunization with several vaccines. They had been vaccinated frequently with both routine and experimental vaccines to protect them from the hazards of working with dangerous germs. Seventy-seven of these workers received an average of more than 190 injections of 21 different vaccines. These highly immunized workers were compared with 26 workers at the same lab who had not received special immunizations. At follow-up intervals of 10, 16 and 25 years, there were *no* important differences in medical history, physical examination or laboratory tests. There was no evidence of increased rates of cancer, immune disorders or death in the highly immunized group.

Passive immunity: Another way to short-term immunity

Passive immunity refers to antibodies that are received from another person, not made by the body's own immune system.

Maternal antibody

Nature provides passive immunity to newborn babies. A mother passes her antibodies to a developing fetus during pregnancy, providing much-needed protection during her newborn's first weeks or months of life. Maternal antibodies vary in amount depending on the mother's levels, and if she has no antibodies against a certain infection, there are none to pass to her baby. Therefore, newborn antibody levels to different germs vary greatly, from one germ to another and from one mother to another.

After birth, an infant's metabolic system gradually breaks down and eliminates these antibodies, which are not replaced unless the infant is exposed to either a germ or a vaccine. Either one will stimulate the infant's own immune system to respond.

For some germs, the amount of antibody passed from mother to infant is not enough to protect the newborn. For such infections it is important to protect the infant by immunizing at a very young age. For other infections, where all mothers have enough antibodies to protect infants for some months, a vaccine may be given later.

Babies born very prematurely are special cases

Most transfer of antibodies from mother to fetus occurs late in pregnancy. Infants born before 26 weeks' gestation get almost no antibody from their mothers and are extremely vulnerable to infection.

What about breast milk?

Breast milk can provide protection against some infections, especially viral respiratory infections, ear infections and some diarrheal infections, but it is no substitute for infant vaccination. The protection provided by

Breast milk's protective effects are limited

Breast milk does not provide enough immunity to protect against the germs for which vaccines are given in infancy. And breast milk only contains antibodies against infections to which the mother herself is immune!

breast milk is incomplete, temporary and can be overcome if the baby is exposed to large amounts of a specific germ.

Antibody injections

In urgent cases, antibodies already produced by a donor are given by injection. This happens in only a few situations:
- To neutralize a toxin, when waiting for a sick person's own immune system to act would be fatal (e.g., in cases of tetanus or diphtheria infection).
- To inactivate a germ before it can cause disease, such as when a non-immune person at high risk for severe disease has been exposed (e.g., to hepatitis B, hepatitis A, measles or chickenpox).
- In people with a condition or having a treatment that prevents the immune system from working. They may be given immune globulin, a blood product containing antibodies to a large number of germs.

Where do these antibodies come from?

They almost always come from human volunteer blood donors who have been thoroughly tested (screened) both for the antibodies that are needed and for any diseases that could be transmitted by blood. The part of blood that contains antibodies (immune globulin) is extracted and concentrated.

One exception is diphtheria antitoxin, which is made in horses.

New ways to make vaccines are being found

Another, newer way to make antibody is used to produce passive immunity to respiratory syncytial virus (RSV). Almost all young babies get an RSV infection early in life, and it can be very serious for babies with certain heart or lung diseases or who are very premature. There is no vaccine for RSV as yet—there may well be in the future—and maternal antibody is not enough to protect the newborn.

Antibody to RSV is made in the laboratory using genetic recombinant techniques to build the antibody molecules. ("Recombinant" means putting genes together.) This form of technology, which avoids the need for living donors—human or horse—will likely be used for other forms of passive immunity in the near future.

Vaccine types

Vaccines differ in how they are made and how they are given. For some vaccines, the whole germ is made inactive (or "killed") in the manufacturing process. For others, parts of the germ which cause the body to make antibodies or T-cells (or both) are extracted and used to make vaccine. For others again, the living germ has been weakened ("attenuated" or modified) in the laboratory to produce a form of the germ that stimulates immunity but does not cause disease.

Inactivated (killed) vaccines. In the early stages of vaccine development, tests are done to determine the amount of antigen needed to cause an immune response. For most vaccines, this amount does not depend on the age or size of the person to be immunized. One exception is hepatitis B vaccine, where higher doses are used in adults and in persons with certain diseases.

Live vaccines. These work differently from inactivated vaccines. They contain a weakened germ which can stimulate the body's immune response without causing disease. A very small amount of the weakened germ is given, usually by injection, although rotavirus vaccine is given by mouth and live influenza vaccine is given by nose spray.

The living germ then multiplies in the body, usually over the next 1 to 3 weeks, producing more antigens and acting enough like the natural infection to cause an immune response.

Live vaccines cause an immune response that closely resembles immunity after natural infection, but inducing this response is a delicate process. For example, if a live vaccine is not stored properly, the vaccine germ can die and the vaccine will not work. Also, if the person being vaccinated already has antibody against the germ, the vaccine germ will be destroyed before it can activate an immune response. This is what happens when a baby is given a live vaccine too early in life, when maternal antibodies are still present (see "Passive immunity", above). Inactivation of the vaccine germ also occurs when someone gets a live vaccine too soon after an injection of antibody, immune globulin or other blood product.

Is there ever a risk of catching the illness from the vaccine itself?

Inactivated vaccines and **purified vaccines** *do not* have any living germs in them, and *cannot* cause infection.

Live attenuated (or weakened) vaccines *do* infect cells and multiply in the body. The vaccine viruses have been weakened in the laboratory, enough that they stimulate immunity without causing a full-blown infection. While they do not cause disease in healthy people, they may occasionally cause disease in people with a condition that has suppressed their immune system severely, and are therefore not given to them. For more information, see Chapter 3, When extra protection is needed.

The table below lists different types of vaccines that you may read about in later chapters.

Table 4.1
Types of vaccines

Type of vaccine	Examples*
Inactivated (killed), intact virus	Polio vaccine, hepatitis A vaccine
Inactivated (killed), fragments of virus	Influenza vaccine
Inactivated bacterial toxin	Diphtheria and tetanus toxoids
Purified viral protein	Hepatitis B vaccine, human papillomavirus vaccine
Purified bacterial proteins	Acellular pertussis vaccine
Purified bacterial polysaccharide (complex sugar)	*Haemophilus influenzae* type b (Hib), pneumococcal, meningococcal and typhoid** vaccines
Live attenuated (weakened) virus	Measles, mumps, rubella, chickenpox vaccines. Oral rotavirus vaccines Intranasal influenza vaccine
Live attenuated (weakened) bacteria	Oral typhoid vaccine**

* Given by injection unless stated otherwise
** Given only for foreign travel

Combination vaccines

You may have noticed in Chapter 2, Routine vaccines, that many vaccines are "combination" vaccines, meaning they contain a number of different vaccines in one shot. Giving these vaccines at the same time *does not* increase the rate of side effects, with one exception: the combined measles-mumps-rubella-varicella (chickenpox) vaccine causes fever more often than the combination measles-mumps-rubella vaccine, with varicella given separately (for more information, see Chapter 6). Also, the protection achieved by a combination vaccine is as effective as by giving the vaccines as separate injections, while reducing the number of shots a child needs.

Vaccine additives

Sometimes, substances are added to vaccines to help ensure their effectiveness and safety. What follows here is a general description of each additive, and why it is used.

> **Vaccine additives may be used:**
> - To support the growth of the bacteria or viruses needed to make the vaccine
> - To inactivate bacteria or viruses
> - As part of the purification process
> - To maintain the stability of the vaccine
> - To enhance vaccine effectiveness

Most of the important additives used are described below. Others include simple salts, sugars and other inert substances.

If you have concerns about additives and your child's allergies, speak with your health care provider.

Preservatives may be added to vaccines in very small amounts to prevent bacterial or fungal contamination. This is necessary when the vaccine is provided in a multi-dose vial that may be opened several times over the period of a month or so. Most vaccines used in Canada today are provided in single-dose vials or pre-filled syringes, where the vaccine remains sterile until used.

- **Thimerosal.** None of the vaccines now made in Canada for routine use in children contain thimerosal. It is present in some brands of hepatitis B and influenza vaccine dispensed in multi-dose vials, which are mainly used when large numbers of people are being vaccinated at the same time. Thimerosal was used in many vaccines from the 1930s until 2001.

  The amount of thimerosal in past vaccines was 100 parts per million. There is *no evidence* that thimerosal caused any form of brain damage when it was used, though public concern was strong. Thimerosal turns into ethylmercury in the body and is rapidly eliminated, so it does not accumulate.

  Thimerosal is often confused with methylmercury, which does accumulate in the body and, in sufficient concentrations, can cause severe brain damage. Methylmercury has never been used in vaccines. The brain damage caused by methylmercury is distinct and very different from autism, attention-deficit disorder or speech and language delay.

  The Institute of Medicine in the United States reviewed all available evidence on the potential toxicity of thimerosal in vaccines and found no evidence of damage caused by this product. Nevertheless, thimerosal was removed from childhood vaccines because of parental concerns.

  Routine vaccines used for children in Canada are thimerosal-free

  But there is no evidence that thimerosal caused any form of brain damage when it was used in vaccines the past.

- **Phenoxyethanol** and **phenol** are two other preservatives that may be present in very tiny amounts in some vaccines, sometimes as traces left from the manufacturing process. Phenoxyethanol is a common preservative in skin creams, perfumes, cosmetics and toothpastes. Phenol, also known as carbolic acid, is used in some antiseptic mouthwashes and in household antiseptics and disinfectants. In high concentrations, far above the trace amounts found in vaccines, these substances may be toxic.

Adjuvants are substances that are added to vaccines to strengthen the immune response.

- **Aluminum** is present as aluminum salts (alum) in vaccines for diphtheria, Hib, hepatitis A, hepatitis B, pertussis, polio, tetanus and in one form of human papillomavirus (HPV) vaccine (Gardasil), in amounts of about 0.3 mg per dose. Aluminum is found in air, food and water and is present in breast milk and infant formula in larger amounts than in any vaccine. Common forms of antacids contain 200 mg to 400 mg of aluminum salts per tablet. Hundreds of millions of people have been safely vaccinated with aluminum-containing vaccines.

- **AS04** is found in one form of HPV vaccine (Cervarix). It contains a substance derived from the cell walls of bacteria combined with aluminum hydroxide.

- **MF59** is present in one form of inactivated influenza vaccine (Fluad). It contains squalene, a naturally occurring substance found in humans, animals and plants. In animals, squalene is made in the liver.

Other substances

- **Antibiotics** are used in some vaccines to prevent bacterial contamination during the manufacturing process. Trace amounts may remain after the purification stage. The types of antibiotics that are most likely to cause a serious allergic reaction (such as penicillin) are *not* contained in vaccines. Traces of kanamycin, neomycin, polymyxin b or streptomycin may be found in vaccines for chickenpox, diphtheria, Hib, hepatitis A, hepatitis B, influenza, measles, mumps, pertussis, polio, rubella, shingles and tetanus. Traces of gentamicin may be found in the intranasal influenza vaccine.

- **Bovine (cow) albumin**, a water-soluble protein, is sometimes used in the production process and traces may be found in some infant combined vaccines, one brand of rotavirus vaccine (RotaTeq), one brand of chickenpox vaccine (Varivax III), and one brand of hepatitis A vaccine (Vaqta). Bovine albumin is obtained only from animals known to be free of disease.

- **Carrier proteins** are chemically linked (or "conjugated") with polysaccharide antigens to produce vaccines that work in infants. Tetanus toxoid is the carrier protein used in Hib vaccines and in two brands of meningococcal vaccine (NeisVac-C and Nimenrix). Diphtheria toxoid is used in the other meningococcal vaccines and in the conjugate pneumococal vaccine (Prevnar13). The amounts of these carrier proteins are too low to stimulate an immune response to tetanus or diphtheria, but may be enough to cause an allergic reaction in someone who has previously had a life-threatening allergic reaction to tetanus or diphtheria vaccine.

- **Egg proteins** may be present in very small amounts in influenza vaccines, which are grown in hens' eggs. Almost all egg protein is removed during the manufacturing process. Vaccinating egg-allergic people with inactivated influenza vaccine in specialized clinics has shown that the yearly flu vaccine can be given safely without any special precautions, other than those used when any vaccine is given. The intranasal (live) form of influenza vaccine has not yet been tested in people with egg allergy, so it is not given at this time to people with a serious egg allergy.

  There has been concern that traces of egg protein may be found in measles and mumps vaccines. But these are produced in chicken cell cultures, not in eggs. Studies have shown that people with an egg allergy have *not* had severe allergic reactions when given these vaccines. Most allergic reactions to measles and mumps vaccines are caused by gelatin or neomycin.

- **Formaldehyde** is used in certain vaccines to kill the virus or bacteria used to make the vaccine, or to inactivate toxins. It is almost all removed during the manufacturing process. Any trace amounts that may remain in the vaccine are safe. Traces of formaldehyde may be present in vaccines for diphtheria, Hib, hepatitis A, hepatitis B, influenza, pertussis, polio and tetanus.

Formaldehyde is produced naturally in the human body and helps with metabolism. There is about 10 times the amount of formaldehyde in an infant's body at any given time than there is in one dose of vaccine.

- **Gelatin** is used as a stabilizing agent in one brand of inactivated influenza vaccine (Fluzone) and in the live intranasal influenza vaccine, as well as in one brand of measles, mumps, rubella vaccine (MMR II), one brand of chickenpox vaccine (Varivax III) and shingles vaccine. Gelatin rarely causes a serious allergic reaction (about one case per 2 million doses). People with a history of life-threatening allergic reactions to gelatin need to be referred to an allergist before receiving these vaccines.

- **Latex** may be present in the stopper at the end of the plunger of pre-filled syringes used for some infant combination vaccines (Boostrix, Infanrix hexa), one brand of hepatitis A vaccine (Havrix), combined hepatitis A and B vaccine (Twinrix), one brand of HPV vaccine (Cervarix) and one brand of meningococcal vaccine (Menjugate). Latex may be present in the vial stoppers of one brand of meningococcal vaccine (Meningitec) and one hepatitis B vaccine (Recombivax).

- **Yeast protein** is used in the production of a few vaccines. Trace amounts may be found in hepatitis B vaccine, combination vaccines containing hepatitis B, and one form of HPV (Gardasil). Serious allergy to yeast is extremely rare.

No vaccine contains human or animal cells, tissue or blood

Human and animal cell cultures are used in the early stages of production of some live vaccines, but **all cells are removed** during purification of the vaccine.

For more detailed information on vaccine components, see the Public Health Agency of Canada's *Canadian Immunization Guide* at www. phac-aspc.gc.ca.

Getting the shot

How vaccines are given

Most vaccines are injected into muscle. In children younger than a year old, they are usually injected into a thigh muscle because it is relatively large. In older children, vaccines are usually given into muscle of the upper arm. Measles, mumps, rubella and chickenpox vaccines, and the polysaccharide pneumococcal vaccine, may also be given by injection into the tissue just under the skin (subcutaneously).

Vaccines against diphtheria, tetanus, pertussis, polio, Hib or hepatitis B and hepatitis A vaccine are injected into muscle rather than subcutaneously because injecting into muscle causes a milder local reaction and the vaccines may work better.

Special care is taken when immunizing people with bleeding disorders, including those receiving anticoagulant drugs. A small gauge needle is used and pressure is applied for 5 to 10 minutes after the shot is given.

Rotavirus vaccine and some travel vaccines are given by mouth. Live influenza vaccine is given as a nose spray. It is likely that in the future, more vaccines will be given by methods other than injection, to minimize pain.

Most vaccines are given in a volume of 0.5 mL (about one-tenth of a teaspoon).

Minimizing pain and discomfort: What to do

Read on to find out what you can do to relieve normal and mild reactions such as pain, fussiness and fever.

Anxiety, stress, fainting

For young children, you can lower stress by breastfeeding, giving sugar water, holding a child close in your arms, staying calm yourself and using distractions (singing, talking, toys). For older children, using the last two strategies and stroking a child's arm before, during and after the needle may help. Sometimes a topical anaesthetic is used to lessen injection pain.

Some adolescents and adults faint when they are anxious or in pain. Their stress can be reduced by a shorter wait time, a comfortable room temperature and privacy during the procedure. To avoid injuries from fainting, people should be immunized while seated or lying down. People who are likely to faint should remain sitting or lying down until they feel better. There are no adverse consequences to fainting, unless an injury occurs by falling. For detailed advice on pain reduction, see the parent guides at the end of this chapter.

Crying, fussiness

Children usually cry and may continue to fuss after getting a shot because of pain at the injection site. In infants, crying with breath-holding spells are a common response to pain.

If your child is crying a lot or is very fussy, you can give acetaminophen, which helps to reduce pain and fever. Some brand names of acetaminophen are Tylenol, Tempra, and Panadol. Ibuprofen (e.g., Advil and Motrin) may be used if a child is over 6 months old and drinking fluids regularly. Use the doses and intervals recommended by your doctor, nurse or pharmacist or as directed on the package.

> **Do not give aspirin (acetylsalicylic acid or ASA) to a child or teen with a fever**
>
> If the fever is due to chickenpox or influenza, aspirin can increase the risk of Reye's syndrome, a very serious condition that may damage the liver and brain.

Be sure to call your child's doctor if crying or fussiness lasts more than 24 hours.

Pain and swelling

If the injection site on your child's leg or arm is swollen, hot, red and/or tender to touch, try these tips to relieve discomfort:
- Apply a clean, cool, wet cloth for 15 to 20 minutes over the sore area.
- Give acetaminophen or ibuprofen. Call your child's doctor or the clinic where the vaccine was given if redness or tenderness continues to worsen 24 hours after it started.

Fever

Children may also develop fever after vaccination but a high fever (above 39°C) is unusual with any of the current vaccines.

If you think your child has a fever, don't guess: check your child's temperature. The most accurate way to do this in a young child is by taking a rectal temperature. Be sure to use a lubricant, such as petroleum jelly, when doing so. Children over 5 years old are usually able to have their temperature taking orally (by mouth). Digital thermometers are preferred to glass mercury thermometers for safety reasons.

To reduce fever:
- Give your child plenty to drink.
- Clothe your child lightly: no extra covers or tight wrappings

You don't always need medication for fever. If your child is uncomfortable, you may give acetaminophen or ibuprofen.

Call the doctor—regardless of how high the fever is—if you are concerned about persistent fever or an unexpected change in your child's behaviour.

Keeping vaccinations—and your child's record—up-to-date

After your child or any family member gets a shot, be sure that you are given a written record of the date and vaccine received. Store vaccination records in a safe place and keep them up-to-date. Don't forget to take this record with you whenever you visit your child's doctor or a health clinic.

Vaccination schedules vary somewhat in different parts of Canada. Decisions about schedules are made by provincial or territorial health authorities based on information about local disease patterns. All schedules used in Canada work well.

Families who move to another part of Canada may miss out on a vaccine because of a regional difference in age at which a vaccine is given. Vaccines that were missed should be given as soon as possible, but there is usually no need to repeat a previous dose, even if the next dose is delayed for a long time.

There is also some regional variation in terms of which vaccines are given free-of-charge and the criteria for providing free vaccines.

If your family is moving...

... to a different province or territory, be sure to take your vaccine records with you. Consult a doctor or clinic in your new location in case the schedule there is different, so no one in the family misses a dose or vaccine because of the move.

Parent guides for reducing vaccination pain and fear in babies, children and adolescents have been developed by The Help ELiminate Pain in KIDS (HELPinKIDS) team at the University of Toronto and adapted by Immunize Canada from the "Clinical Practice Guideline: Reducing the pain of childhood vaccination: an evidence-based clinical practice guideline" CMAJ 2010;182(18):E843-E855, and reproduced here with the kind permission of the Canadian Medical Association. Illustrated versions of these documents can be freely downloaded at http://immunize.ca/uploads/iaw/2013/3p_babiesto1yr_e.pdf and http://immunize.ca/uploads/pain/3p_kidsandteens_e.pdf.

Reduce the pain of vaccination in babies: A guide for parents

Why is vaccination pain a concern?
- Vaccinations are a routine part of baby's medical care. They protect a baby from serious diseases.
- Most babies experience pain from vaccinations. Pain can cause a baby to develop a fear of doctors, nurses and needles.
- No parent wants to see a baby in pain. Some parents delay or stop vaccinations because of pain. This can leave a baby without protection from serious diseases.

Plan ahead
- Below are methods that you can use to reduce your baby's pain during vaccinations. These methods are proven to be safe and effective. **You can combine the different methods for better results**.
- Plan what you will do for your baby's next vaccination. Tell your baby's health care provider so they can support your goals.
- Bring your baby's vaccination record, and pack any supplies you will need in your baby's diaper bag.
- After your baby's vaccination, judge how much pain your baby had. Observe your baby's:
  – body movements (calm or thrashing?),
  – facial expressions (neutral or locked in grimace?),
  – sounds (silent or high-pitched cry?).
- Use what you see to plan what you will do the next time to reduce your baby's pain.
- To see a video, visit Immunize Canada at http://immunize.ca/en/parents/pain.aspx

What you can do
Breastfeed your baby
- Undress your baby to free the leg(s) or arm(s) where the vaccination needle(s) will be given before you start breastfeeding.

- Start to breastfeed your baby **before** the vaccination needle. Make sure you have a good latch. Then continue breastfeeding **during and after** the vaccination needle. Breastfeeding your baby during the vaccination needle combines holding, sweet taste and sucking, and may promote calmness.
- Breastfeeding during the vaccination needle is safe for babies, even newborns. *There is no evidence that babies will choke or associate their mother with pain.*
- If you are not breastfeeding your baby during vaccination needle(s), bottle feed your baby with expressed breast milk or formula and hold your baby **before, during and after** the vaccination needle. This will simulate aspects of breastfeeding.

Hold your baby

- If you are not breastfeeding your baby during vaccination needle(s), you can hold your baby to reduce pain.
- Undress your baby to free the leg(s) or arm(s) where the vaccination needle(s) will be given.
- Then position your baby upright and hold your baby close **before, during and after** the vaccination needle.
  - You can sit on a chair or lean against the examination table to minimize the risk for accidental falls.
  - If your baby is a month old or less, you can place your baby against your chest.
- Holding your baby helps your baby to feel secure and to stay still. Don't hold your baby too tightly. If you do, your baby may get upset.
- You may gently pat or rock your baby **after** the vaccination needle.

How you can act

Your state of mind

- Stay with your baby **before, during and after** vaccination needles. Try to be calm, use your normal speaking voice, and be positive. This will help your baby stay calm. Babies see and feel what their parents are doing, and often do the same.

- If you are nervous, you can take a few slow breaths to calm yourself. Breathe so your belly expands, not your chest. You can do this while holding your baby.

What you can give

Topical anaesthetic cream, gel or patch

- Topical anaesthetics reduce the pain from vaccination needles. In Canada, there are 3 different brands you can buy from a drug store without a prescription: EMLA™ (lidocaine-prilocaine), Ametop™(tetracaine), and Maxilene™(lidocaine).
- These products dull pain where the vaccination needle enters your baby's skin.
- They are safe for babies, even newborns.
- It is recommended that you apply them at home or as soon as you arrive at the clinic because you will have to wait for them to take effect. Leave them on the skin undisturbed for the recommended waiting time: 60 minutes for EMLA™; 45 minutes for Ametop™; and 30 minutes for Maxilene™.
- Talk with your baby's health care provider about how to apply them. For babies under 1 year of age, they are usually applied to the upper outer part of the leg; for children aged 1 year and older, they are usually applied to the upper arm. If your baby is getting more than one needle, apply to both legs or both arms.
- If using the patch, just peel off the backing and stick the patch on the skin. If using the cream or gel, squeeze out 1 g (about the size of a 5-cent coin) on the skin and cover it with the dressing provided or with plastic wrap.
- Remove the medicine after the waiting time. Your baby's skin may appear whiter or redder than normal. This is okay and will go away.
- Allergic skin reactions are rare. If there is a rash, talk to your baby's health care provider about it. It could be an allergic skin reaction.

Sucrose solution

- If you are not breastfeeding your baby during your baby's vaccination needle(s), you can use sucrose solution (also known as sugar water) to reduce your baby's pain. Sucrose solution is safe for babies, even newborns. It is included as a flavouring agent in other medications commonly used in babies such as antibiotics and fever medications.

- You can make sucrose solution at home or at the clinic by mixing 1 teaspoon of white sugar with 2 teaspoons boiled water. For babies over 6 months, you may use tap water if the tap water is safe for drinking.
- Give your baby some sucrose solution 1 to 2 minutes **before** the vaccination needle.
- Use a dropper (or syringe) and place the sucrose solution into the side of your baby's mouth between the cheeks and gums. Give your baby one drop at a time and let your baby suck on the sweet taste.
- You may also dip a soother into the sucrose solution water and give it to your baby **during** the vaccination needle. Combining sucrose solution with a soother and holding your baby can simulate aspects of breastfeeding.
- Sugar water should not be used to calm a crying baby at home. Parents who are thinking about introducing a soother should talk to their health care provider about the possible effects soothers can have on breastfeeding and oral health.

Reduce the pain of vaccination in kids and teens: A guide for parents

Why is vaccination pain a concern?
- Vaccinations are a routine part of a child's medical care. They offer protection from serious diseases.
- Most vaccines are given with a needle. This can be painful and frightening for children.
- Some parents and children delay or stop vaccinations because of pain and fear. This can leave children without protection from serious diseases.

Plan ahead to reduce pain
- Below are methods that you can use to reduce pain during vaccinations. These methods are proven to be safe and effective. You can combine the different methods for better results.
- Plan what you will do for your child's next vaccination. Tell your child's health care provider so they can help you.
- With children three years of age and older talk ahead of time about what will happen, how it will feel and what you will do to manage discomfort.
- After your child's vaccination, judge how much pain your child had. You can observe your child's body movements (calm or thrashing?), face (normal or locked in a grimace?), and sounds (silent or high-pitched cry?).
- Children three years of age and older can report their own pain. Use what your child tells you and what you see to plan what you will do to reduce your child's vaccination pain the next time.
- To see a video, visit Immunize Canada at http://immunize.ca/en/parents/pain.aspx .

What you can give
Topical anaesthetics

- Topical anaesthetics reduce the pain from vaccination needles. In Canada, there are 3 different brands you can buy from a drug store without a prescription: EMLA™ (lidocaine-prilocaine), Ametop™ (tetracaine), and Maxilene™ (lidocaine).
- These products dull pain where the vaccination needle enters your child's skin. They are safe for children of all ages.
- It is recommended that you apply them at home or as soon as you arrive at the clinic because you will have to wait for them to take effect. Leave them on the skin undisturbed for the recommended waiting time: 60 minutes for EMLA™; 45 minutes for Ametop™; and 30 minutes for Maxilene™. Talk with your child's health care provider about how to apply them.
- Topical anaesthetics are usually applied to the upper arm. Confirm the location with your child's health care provider. If your child is getting more than one vaccination needle, apply to both arms.
- If using the patch, just peel off the backing and stick the patch on the skin. If using the cream or gel, squeeze out 1 g (about the size of a 5-cent coin) on the skin and cover it with the dressing provided or with plastic wrap.
- Remove the medicine after the waiting time. Your child's skin may appear whiter or redder than normal. This is okay and will go away.
- Allergic skin reactions are rare. If there is a rash, talk to your child's health care provider about it. It could be an allergic skin reaction.

What you can do
Upright positioning

- Undress your child to free the arm(s) where the vaccination needle(s) will be given.

- Have your child sit upright **before, during, and after** the vaccination needle(s). Your child may be held on your lap. This helps your child to feel secure and to stay still.
- *Don't hold too tightly—if you do, this can increase your child's distress.*

How you can act
Your state of mind
- Stay with your child, be calm and use your normal speaking voice **before, during and after** vaccination needle(s).
- *Don't use words that focus attention on the vaccination needle or pain such as: "it'll be over soon" or "here comes the sting" and don't lie to your child about how it will feel: "it doesn't hurt".*
- Do use neutral words and stay positive: "Here we go" or "you did great". This will help your child stay calm.
- Children see and feel what their parents are doing, and often do the same. If you are nervous, you can take a few slow breaths to calm yourself. Breathe so your belly expands, not your chest.

Distract your child
- Taking your child's focus away from the vaccination needle(s) can reduce your child's pain.
- Distract your child with bubbles, pinwheels, music or videos. You may use electronic devices like smartphones and tablets.
- For best results, choose a distraction that involves multiple senses and have your child actively participate. The more involved your child is in the distraction, the better it will work.
- Be prepared to change what you are doing to keep your child distracted.
- *There are a few children that cope better if they watch the vaccination needle(s), so if your child says they want to watch, that's okay too.*

5

Vaccine safety and effectiveness

Most parents know that vaccines are tested before they can be given to the general public. But they are probably less aware of the extensive monitoring, testing, information-sharing and decision-making that goes on behind the scenes.

All year round, year after year, knowledgeable people keep a watchful eye on any side effects and reactions following vaccination, as well as on the diseases these vaccines prevent.

Vaccines, like medicines, must go through a series of steps before they are approved for use. Before any vaccine is approved for use in Canada, it must be shown to be safe and effective in preventing the disease that it targets. Vaccines are among the most strictly regulated medical products in Canada.

This chapter looks at the systems in place to ensure the safety and effectiveness of vaccines. The large network of professionals, committees and organizations monitoring infectious diseases and vaccines in Canada is described. Their role is to oversee the testing, safety and effectiveness of vaccines, as well as to make recommendations on best practice. Their recommendations are based on extensive knowledge of diseases and vaccines. Unlike some other sources of information, these experts can be trusted to make sound decisions based on the most up-to-date and credible information.

Later in this chapter we describe how scientists interpret the results of tests for vaccine safety (i.e., Are there any side effects?) and effectiveness (i.e., Does the vaccine do what it is supposed to?).

Ensuring vaccine safety

Health authorities in Canada, including those in provincial and federal governments, take vaccine safety very seriously. Before a vaccine is licensed for use in Canada, the manufacturer must prove that their product is safe. This is done with studies to compare the immune and other reactions of people who are given the vaccine with those in people who are given an injection which does not contain the vaccine. People taking part in these studies (or "trials") are volunteers. They understand that a vaccine is being studied and are informed about the possible side effects that may occur.

Monitoring vaccine safety is ongoing

Trials carried out before a vaccine is licensed can show that serious adverse effects after getting the vaccine being tested are uncommon. But because of the limited number of participants, such trials may not pick up the possibility of rare adverse effects.

Monitoring for possible but rare serious adverse events must continue after any vaccine has been licensed for use.

The **Biologics and Genetic Therapies Directorate (BGTD)**, which is part of Health Canada, regulates vaccines used in humans in Canada. They approve vaccines for use only if all acceptable standards of quality, safety and efficacy are met. The BGTD also supervises all aspects of production and quality control throughout the vaccine's life cycle, ensuring that the batches used to immunize children today are as safe and effective as the ones tested during original clinical trials. The factory where a vaccine is manufactured is inspected by government authorities at regular intervals to ensure that facilities and all stages of production and quality control conform to the highest standards.

Each individual batch of vaccine must also be authorized for sale in Canada. Manufacturers have to submit an official document providing results from all the tests for quality performed throughout the production process for that batch. Also, for most vaccines, the BGTD performs tests on samples from each batch in its own laboratory to monitor vaccine quality.

Monitoring vaccine safety

After BGTD has approved a vaccine, Canada has advanced systems in place to monitor safety and to make our medical experts aware of unusual post-vaccine events. In the very rare event that a batch of vaccine results in an unexpected side effect, these systems can ensure that the rest of the batch is not used. Canada is—and has been for a while—a world leader in post-marketing surveillance of vaccine adverse events.

What *is* an adverse event?

An adverse event following immunization (AEFI) is any "untoward medical occurance" after a vaccine has been given which may—or may not—have been caused by the vaccination. Some mild reactions are **expected**, such as fever and redness, swelling and soreness at an injection site.

An **unexpected** AEFI is one that was not recognized previously and was not listed in information supplied by the manufacturer.

A **serious** AEFI is one that is life-threatening and/or results in hospitalization, permanent disability, or death.

Voluntary reporting by health care professionals

In all provinces and territories, doctors and public health nurses are expected to report any *serious* or *unexpected* AEFI that occurs after vaccination to their local health department, especially if it is serious enough to require a visit to a doctor or hospitalization. Many less serious and expected events, such as fever or local reactions (e.g., redness, swelling) are also reported, especially if these occur in clusters or more frequently than usual.

- The local medical officer of health investigates all of these reports, then forwards them to the provincial or territorial ministry of health.
- The reports then go to the Canadian Adverse Events Following Immunization Surveillance System (CAEFISS), a branch of the Public Health Agency of Canada. This federal agency keeps track of, and analyzes, all reports of adverse events after vaccination. CAEFISS receives about 4,000 reports each year. However, most reports concern minor adverse events such as fever or a local reaction (e.g., redness, swelling).

Mandatory reporting by manufacturers

All vaccine manufacturers must report promptly any serious adverse events that they become aware of, in Canada or internationally, to Health Canada.

IMPACT

Canada has a unique program called IMPACT—the Canadian Immunization Monitoring Program, ACTive—to detect adverse events related to vaccination and monitor vaccine-preventable diseases. The program is funded by the Public Health Agency of Canada and operated by the Canadian Paediatric Society.

IMPACT was designed over 20 years ago by researchers at paediatric health centres in Canada who were interested in vaccination. The program works as follows:

- A nurse at each of 12 children's hospitals across Canada reviews all admissions to the hospital for certain serious illnesses, including seizures, encephalitis, encephalopathy, loss of consciousness,

meningitis, acute paralysis, bleeding or bruising, some types of rashes, and severe allergic reactions. Each year, these nurses screen more than 100,000 admissions at the 12 hospitals.
• If a child with any of these diagnoses had recently received a vaccine, a report is sent to the local health department and to CAEFISS for analysis.

IMPACT has been operating since 1991

Through the years, this program has collected much-needed data on the safety of vaccines.

For example, IMPACT has confirmed that severe neurologic (brain) illness following vaccination is an extremely rare occurrence. Cases of encephalitis, encephalopathy, acute paralysis or other brain damage are extremely rare, and the role of vaccine in individual cases is often questionable.

For more information, see: www.cps.ca/en/impact

CPSP

With the Canadian Paediatric Surveillance Program (CPSP), Canada has another valuable and unique surveillance tool for collecting active real-time data on rare diseases, including acute paralysis in children and some vaccine-preventable diseases.

The CPSP was established in 1996 through a partnership between the Public Health Agency of Canada and the Canadian Paediatric Society. The program involves more than 2,500 paediatricians and paediatric subspecialists from all provinces and territories who monitor their practices for rare conditions and report monthly to the CPSP.

CPSP surveillance of acute flaccid paralysis enabled Canada to fulfill its international obligations to the Pan American Health Organization and the World Health Organization by demonstrating the absence of paralytic polio and wild polioviruses in Canada.

For more information about the CPSP, see: www.cpsp.cps.ca

Public Health Agency of Canada

Experts with this government body review all reported cases of serious adverse events following vaccination that result in hospitalization, permanent damage or death. Included for review are all cases of meningitis, encephalitis, encephalopathy, seizures without fever, death, or any event that required hospitalization following immunization.

Because such events are not necessarily caused by vaccination but may be linked in time by coincidence, careful review of the details of all cases, on a regular basis, is important to determine whether there are any concerns regarding vaccine safety.

The results of these reviews are reported to the doctor or nurse who reported the event. Summaries of results are posted on the Public Health Agency of Canada's website under Vaccine Safety: www.phac-aspc.gc.ca/im/vs-sv/index-eng.php

Global Advisory Committee on Vaccine Safety

The World Health Organization established this committee in 1999 to advise on vaccine safety issues of potential global importance. The committee members are acknowledged experts from around the world in the fields of epidemiology (the study of disease incidence, control and prevention), statistics, paediatrics, internal medicine, pharmacology and toxicology, infectious diseases, public health, immunology and autoimmunity, and drug regulation and safety. This committee has reviewed almost all issues relating to vaccine safety. Reports of the committee's reviews are available at: www.who.int/vaccine_safety/committee/topics/en/

Immunization Safety Review Committee

The Institute of Medicine (IOM) in the United States formed this committee to evaluate all available evidence on various immunization safety concerns. Specifically, the committee was asked to present its findings regarding possible causal associations between vaccines and certain adverse outcomes. Comprised of experts in infectious diseases, immunization, epidemiology, statistics and public health, the committee reviewed relevant published scientific and medical articles as well as unpublished data, personal communications and submissions by any interested parties. Their conclusions and recommendations are published by the National Academy of Sciences in eight reports, which can be downloaded at no cost from the Institute of Medicine's website at: www.iom.edu/

The system works! Responses to safety monitoring

- In the late 1980s, an increased rate of meningitis was noted after a new strain of mumps vaccine was introduced in Canada. The vaccine was withdrawn.
- Oral (live) polio vaccine is very effective in controlling polio and was used in Canada when polio was still being transmitted in this country. However, in extremely rare cases (about 1 in 2.4 million doses) this form of vaccine caused paralysis. Once polio was brought under control in North America, the live vaccine was no longer used. It was replaced by an inactivated vaccine.
- In 2000-01, there were reports of a new oculo-respiratory syndrome (red eyes, cough and difficulty breathing) after influenza vaccine. Although these symptoms were mild and cleared within 48 hours in most cases, investigations were made to determine the cause. Changes to the vaccine manufacturing process have made this syndrome very rare.

Ensuring vaccine effectiveness

Before a vaccine is licensed for use in Canada, its manufacturers must prove that their product prevents the disease it is directed against. This is done by determining the number of cases of the disease in individuals who have received the vaccine and the number of disease cases in unvaccinated individuals. When the disease is rare, the ability of immunized people to develop antibodies against the infection may be used to indicate vaccine effectiveness.

After a vaccine has been licensed for use, monitoring for new cases of the infection is carried out to determine whether the vaccine continues to be effective. Health care professionals must report all cases of selected infections to their local public health authorities. This information is then forwarded to the provincial or territorial ministry of health and from there to the Public Health Agency of Canada's Notifiable Disease Surveillance System.

The **IMPACT** program (see "Vaccine safety", above) also reviews hospital admissions for certain vaccine-preventable diseases and reports these to the IMPACT data centre and the Public Health Agency of Canada for analysis. This program has collected data to assess the effects of vaccination programs on selected vaccine-preventable diseases.

The **CPSP** (see "Vaccine safety", above) has also collected much-needed data on several vaccine-preventable diseases and their consequences, such as congenital rubella syndrome (rubella in early pregnancy causes severe malformations in the fetus), necrotizing fasciitis (a serious skin infection that can complicate chickenpox), and subacute sclerosing panencephalitis (a serious complication of measles).

Information about the numbers and rates of infections is used to determine whether the vaccines used are continuing to be effective (that is, doing their job).

Vaccines work

While no vaccine is 100% effective, all vaccines used for the routine immunization of children are highly effective in preventing disease.

In fact, these vaccines are so effective that most of the diseases they protect against are now very rare.

Why do some children who have been vaccinated still get measles?

Opponents of vaccination are quick to point out that many cases of measles occur in vaccinated children. They claim this proves that the vaccine doesn't work. In recent outbreaks of measles in Canada and the United States, some who were immunized earlier still caught measles. But to say that this means the vaccine doesn't work is incorrect.

We know that measles vaccine is not 100% effective. Let's assume that about 1 in 200 (0.5%) of children are not protected after 2 doses of vaccine and use this number in an example.

Example: In a community with 2,000 children, assume that 95% are vaccinated. This means that there are 1900 vaccinated children and 100 unvaccinated children. The number of children who are still susceptible to measles is 100 unvaccinated children plus 0.5% of the 1900 vaccinated children who are unprotected (10), for a total of 110 children.

One child comes home from a trip abroad with measles. Measles is so contagious that it quickly spreads. One-half of the 110 susceptible children catch it: half of the 100 unvaccinated children (or 50) get measles and half of the 10 children whose vaccine failed (or 5) get measles. Therefore, there are 55 cases of measles. The proportion of cases that occurred in vaccinated children is 5 of the total 55, or about one-tenth. This seems very high, *but it does not mean that the vaccine fails one-tenth of the time.*

The 50 cases of measles in the unvaccinated group came from a total of 100 children; the attack rate in this group is 50%. The 5 cases of vaccine failure came from a total of 1900 children, an attack rate of only 0.25%. From these numbers, we can see that unvaccinated children were 200 times more likely to catch measles!

The science of cause and effect

How do scientists determine whether a vaccine causes an adverse event? And how do they determine whether a vaccine prevents disease? The same principles are used to answer both questions.

Since parents are often concerned about the safety of vaccines, the following discussion explains how scientists use different methods to try to answer questions about causes of adverse events seen after vaccination. A simple example has been used to illustrate the different methods.

Temporal vs. causal association. Here's an everyday example. One event, eating ice cream (event A), may be followed by another event, such as sweating (event B). Events that occur in this way are said to have a *temporal* association—they are related to each other in time. This doesn't necessarily mean there is a cause and effect, or **causal** relationship. In other words, the fact that event B follows event A does not mean that A caused B; it may be just a coincidence.

Proof vs. probability. Science cannot prove that one event can *never* cause another. For instance, it cannot prove that eating ice cream (event A) will never make a person sweat (event B). What science *can* determine is the *likelihood* that eating ice cream will make a person sweat. Or, to be more exact, science can determine the *probability* of a particular outcome having occurred by chance.

Imagine that a person did sweat after eating ice cream. Scientists could review all of the circumstances surrounding the event and tell us their findings: it is 99.9% certain that these two events happened by chance —it was the extreme heat that day that made the person sweat, not the ice cream. People are more likely to eat ice cream on a hot day.

In this case, the events of eating the ice cream and sweating are linked in time: there is a temporal association. There is no causal association: the ice cream did not cause the sweating!

A vaccine-related example. A small proportion of babies who have died of sudden infant death syndrome (SIDS) had been vaccinated within a day of dying. Did vaccination cause the death? Many studies have shown that there is no increased risk of SIDS following vaccination. The association between vaccination and SIDS is purely coincidental. It occurs because vaccination is very common in infants between 2 and 6 months old, the time period when most cases of SIDS occur.

By contrast, the association between a baby's sleeping position (event A) and SIDS (event B) *has* been found to be causal: event A causes event B. Babies who sleep on their stomachs are much more likely to die of SIDS than babies who sleep on their backs. Results of the "Back to Sleep" campaign, which was designed to raise awareness about the back-sleep position, confirm the causal association between sleep position and SIDS:

- More than two-thirds of parents now put their babies on their back to sleep in Canada, the United States, the United Kingdom, Australia and New Zealand.
- Since this change, the occurrence rate of SIDS has been cut by more than 50% in these countries and many others as well.

Analyzing data

How do scientists determine whether association is causal or coincidental?

By examining several different kinds of information, scientists can learn whether one event causes another.

Let's use the ice cream and sweating example again.

Close temporal association. Do the two events happen within the same sequence and in the same time period? A temporal association is a necessary condition of cause and effect. But it is not sufficient proof that one event causes the other, since the temporal association could be purely coincidental. To learn whether event B occurs after event A, careful investigation of a number of cases of event B is carried out. In our ice cream example, scientists would review other cases that involved eating ice cream and sweating to determine whether sweating always occurred *after* eating ice cream, or whether, in some cases, it occurred *before*. Other reasons for the sweating—nervousness, a medical condition involving the sweat glands, or eating ice cream while sitting beside a roaring fire—would be explored.

Strength of association. Researchers and scientists perform experimental studies. They compare two groups of subjects to find out the frequency or risk of event B (sweating) in both groups. The experimental group is exposed to event A (they eat ice cream), but the control group is not exposed (they don't eat ice cream). How many people eating ice cream would be sweating? How many people not eating the ice cream would be sweating? The frequency of event B (sweating) in the two groups is compared and analyzed using statistical methods.

The strength of an association is measured in terms of relative risk. For example, let's use the frequency of sweating as our unit of measure. To calculate the relative risk between sweating and eating ice cream, first, we calculate the frequency of sweating in people eating ice cream and in people not eating ice cream. Then, we divide the frequency in those eating ice cream by the frequency in those not eating ice cream.

Relative risk equals 1.0. If the risk is the same for both groups (i.e., 5% of people sweated while eating ice cream and 5% of people sweated while not eating ice cream), the relative risk equals 1.0. In this case, there is no evidence of an increased risk for people eating ice cream, and there is no association between eating ice cream and sweating. Sweating after eating ice cream is a coincidence.

Relative risk greater than 1.0. If the relative risk is greater than 1.0 (i.e., 10% of people sweated while eating ice cream but only 2% sweated in the non-ice cream group with a relative risk of 10/2 = 5.0) then there is evidence of a positive association. In this case, eating ice cream is likely to cause the sweating. The greater the value of the relative risk, the greater the likelihood that the association is causal.

Relative risk less than 1.0. A relative risk of less than 1.0 (i.e., 1% sweated while eating the ice cream but 8% sweated in the non-ice cream group, with a relative risk of 1/8 = 0.125) means that there is no positive association. In this case, ice cream is very likely not to cause the sweating; indeed, it may prevent sweating!

Studying associations between vaccines and adverse events

Epidemiological methods are often used to learn about associations between diseases and their suspected causes, including an adverse event occurring after a vaccine has been given. The frequency of the event is measured in a group given the vaccine and in a group not given the vaccine. If the frequency is the same in both groups (relative risk of 1.0), there is no causal association. Tests of vaccines for safety before they are licensed are done in this way.

A related method can be used once a vaccine has been licensed and is being used in many children, especially if concern is raised about a possible rare adverse event that was not discovered in studies before licensing—e.g., SIDS. Epidemiologists looked at all cases of SIDS in a particular population in a specific time period and determined whether these babies had been vaccinated. They then calculated the proportion of children with SIDS who had been vaccinated and the proportion of a group of children of the same age without SIDS who had been vaccinated. These proportions were the same. Thus, there was no evidence that vaccination caused SIDS: the event was a coincidence.

Other types of information that may be assessed when determining causality

Positive association in animal experimentation. Does event A produce event B in animals in controlled experiments? For example, do animals sweat after eating ice cream in a laboratory? Very early in the stages of development of a new vaccine, safety studies are carried out in animals before similar studies are done in humans.

Unique and specific outcome. Is the outcome or event B (in this case, sweating), a unique and specific reaction that occurs only after the cause in question (event A, eating ice cream) and never at other times? This was the case when oculorespiratory syndrome was linked with some batches of influenza vaccine—the syndrome only happened after the vaccine was given.

Dose–response relationship. To go back to our ice cream example, in a dose–response relationship, suppose that as the amount of ice cream a person eats increases, the risk of sweating also increases. This would indicate that ice cream did cause sweating. For a vaccine, if an event occurred more frequently when a person was given a larger dose—or more doses—of a vaccine, this would suggest that the vaccine caused the event.

Replication of findings. If the association is causal, it should be found consistently in different studies done by different researchers in different places. Put another way, the vaccine should cause that same event in each study.

Alternative explanations. A thorough search for all other causes or risk factors should be made in order to rule out alternative explanations. In the ice cream example, another cause may be the temperature of the place where the ice cream is being eaten.

Cessation of exposure. The frequency of event B (sweating) should decline when exposure to event A (eating ice cream) is reduced or eliminated. The frequency of hypotensive-hyporesponsive attacks in infants, a recognized adverse effect of the old whole-cell pertussis vaccine, dropped dramatically when the vaccine was replaced by a more purified antigen vaccine.

Demonstrable biological mechanism. The process by which event A produces event B should be explainable by information that is credible and known to be true (e.g., the laws of physics, knowledge about the way the digestive system works). In the example being used, researchers would have to find a biological explanation for ice cream causing a person to sweat. Likewise, with an unexpected adverse event following vaccination, a biological mechanism would be sought. When oculorespiratory syndrome with influenza vaccine was first recognized, it was investigated and evidence suggested it was due to an inflammatory reaction to clumps of vaccine particles in some batches of vaccine.

To sum up

Scientific methods are used to determine whether adverse events are caused by a vaccine as well as to show how well vaccines work. A simple example—one that is unrelated to vaccines—has been used to make some of the points in this chapter clearer. Based on all available scientific evidence, the vaccines currently in use have been shown to be extremely safe and effective.

Vaccination has been and still is one of the most important ways to prevent illness and disease. **The benefits of vaccination far outweigh the extremely rare risks of serious adverse events.**

Making recommendations on vaccine use

You may wonder why vaccines are available for some diseases and not for others, and who decides which vaccines to recommend. There are two main reasons for having a vaccine:
- The disease it prevents must be sufficiently serious to make immunization worthwhile, either for the general population or for individuals at higher risk of getting a serious disease or its complications.
- There must be a safe and effective vaccine available.

There are infections causing serious disease in Canada today for which vaccines are not available, though they may be in the near future. Here are some examples:
- Respiratory syncytial virus sends many infants to hospital with severe respiratory infections each year.
- Group B streptococcus causes serious infections in newborn infants.
- Group A streptococcus causes not only strep throat and impetigo, but flesh-eating disease, shock and rheumatic fever.
- Lyme disease, an infection spread by tick bites that causes rash, fever, headache and arthritis, is on the increase in Canada.
- Hepatitis C is another chronic viral infection of the liver.
- HIV is a devastating disease world-wide.

Who decides?

NACI. The Public Health Agency of Canada's National Advisory Committee on Immunization (NACI) makes recommendations on the use of vaccines in Canada. NACI reports to the federal Minister of Health. NACI members are non-governmental experts in infectious diseases, immunization, immunology, epidemiology and public health.

- The committee regularly reviews all the scientific information available on the safety and efficacy of vaccines—new vaccines as well as vaccines already in use.
- Recommendations on vaccine use are posted on the Public Health Agency of Canada's website and published in the *Canada Communicable Disease Report* at: www.phac-aspc.gc.ca/publicat/ ccdr-rmtc/.
- NACI issues updated statements on vaccine safety and use whenever appropriate.
- The committee also publishes the *Canadian Immunization Guide*, available online at: www.phac-aspc.gc.ca/publicat/cig-gci/ index-eng.php. The last paper version of this guide was published in 2006. The online version was completed in 2013 and is updated continually, as soon as new information becomes available.
- NACI also exchanges information with the Public Health Service in the United States. The chair of NACI is a member of the U.S. Advisory Committee on Immunization Practices (ACIP) and attends all of the meetings of that committee. A member of ACIP also attends NACI meetings. This two-way relationship between the Canadian and American committees ensures that members of both are up-to-date with recommendations made by their counterparts and the information on which their decisions are based.

The **Canadian Paediatric Society (CPS) Infectious Diseases and Immunization Committee** makes recommendations about vaccines and immunization programs. Some members are also members of NACI. The chair of this committee acts as liaison with the American Academy of Pediatrics (AAP) Committee on Infectious Diseases, while a member of the AAP also sits on the CPS committee.

CPS recommendations are available in *Paediatrics & Child Health*, the journal of the CPS, and online at: www.cps.ca. Recommendations from the American Academy of Pediatrics are available in *Pediatrics*, the AAP journal, and incorporated into their *Red Book*, a definitive AAP resource on infectious diseases published every three years.

Keeping up-to-date. With so much crossover among committees, all their members—Canadian and American alike—keep up-to-date with vaccine policies and recommendations on this continent and around the world.

The **Canadian Immunization Committee (CIC)** is made up of medical officers of health or their representatives from each province and territory, along with federal government representatives and immunization experts. The CIC considers NACI recommendations and provides analyses of costs and advice on operational and technical issues to aid the provinces and territories in making decisions about their vaccine programs.

Provinces and territories. The final decision on whether to add a new vaccine to a publicly funded immunization program or to change the groups to whom an existing vaccine is given free of charge is made by the government of each province or territory, who also pays for the vaccine. They consider local disease patterns, priorities and available funds. Because of this, vaccine programs are not identical across Canada.

6

Adverse effects and common concerns

We learned in Chapter 4 that some mild adverse events following immunization are both common and expected. This chapter looks at these events or reactions in more detail. Getting a shot isn't a fun experience for a child or parent. But after reading this chapter, you will know when your child is reacting normally to the vaccine experience and when there may be cause for concern. For suggestions on how to help make immunization less stressful for your child, see Chapter 4.

Parents may hear stories about possibly harmful effects of vaccines, either from someone they know or in the media. This chapter also examines and responds to common vaccine fears. Questions often asked by concerned parents are answered here.

Finally, to provide perspective, we compare the risks of routine vaccines with the risks of diseases they protect against. Table 6.1 shows, with specifics, that vaccine-related risks are far, far fewer than those associated with the diseases themselves.

Vaccine side effects: Common and uncommon

Common reactions

- **Injection site reactions.** Redness and pain (with or without swelling), are the most common side effects of any vaccine that is given by injection. Usually these reactions are mild and resolve quickly.
- **Fever and seizures.** Fever often occurs after vaccination and may, in a few cases, cause seizures (convulsions).

Fever-related (or "febrile") seizures are caused by high fever. Fever can trigger a seizure in about 3% of healthy young children and is the most common cause of seizures in children between 6 months and 6 years old. Febrile seizures occur most often when fever is caused by *infection* rather than by a vaccine. They are not dangerous and do not cause brain damage of any kind. However, febrile seizures are more likely to happen in children who already have epilepsy or a brain disorder.

Can vaccines cause seizures?

Yes, indirectly. Vaccines can cause fever, and fever can cause seizures. Therefore, vaccine-induced fever can cause seizures, more often in children whose parents or siblings have also had febrile seizures.

If your child has a febrile seizure, ask your doctor what you should do if it happens again. There is no evidence that medications to reduce fever prevent febrile seizures.

Rare reactions

- **Anaphylaxis** is a serious, potentially life-threatening type of allergic reaction. It usually occurs within minutes of exposure to the source of the allergy, with sudden hives, swelling of the mouth and face, difficulty breathing and a drop in blood pressure. Anaphylaxis can be a reaction to a particular food or medication, and is extremely rare after a vaccine (1 to 10 cases per million doses of vaccine given). If anaphylaxis occurs on the day a vaccine was given, and no other cause for this reaction is found, the child should not be given that specific vaccine again *except* in a special clinic equipped to prevent and control anaphylaxis.

- **Guillain-Barré syndrome**, a form of paralysis, has been reported after influenza vaccine but only rarely, at a rate of about one case per million people vaccinated. There have also been rare reports of this syndrome after other vaccines, though it is not known for sure whether the vaccine is responsible.

Side effects of single component vaccines

For information on other, possible side effects after receiving vaccines with only one component—hepatitis A, hepatitis B, human papillomavirus, influenza, meningococcal, pneumococcal, rotavirus—see the chapters on these infections.

Side effects of combination vaccines

Vaccines containing combinations of diphtheria, tetanus, pertussis, polio, Hib and hepatitis B

Depending on a child's age at the time of vaccination, between three and six of these components may be given together as a single combined vaccine. Getting these components as a combined vaccine does not produce more side effects than getting single component vaccines.

Common reactions:

Injection site (local) reactions (redness, swelling and soreness) are the most common reactions, occurring in 10% to 40% of infants after each of the first 3 doses. Usually, these side effects start within 12 to 24 hours of vaccination, are mild, last 1 to 2 days, and do not affect behaviour, though a child may be fussy.

The likelihood of local reactions increases with the number of doses given. After getting the booster at 4 to 6 years of age, about 1 in 5 children have a larger local reaction, with redness and swelling at the injection site that is larger than 5 cm (2 in.) in size. However, even with these larger reactions, only 1% to 2% of children experience pain that limits arm movement. A few children develop a firm lump at the injection site, which may not appear for days or weeks after vaccination. This lump is caused by inflammation and almost always disappears with time.

Here are a few points to keep in mind:

- Local reactions are much more common in older children and adults receiving booster doses than in children younger than 2 years old.

- Severe local reactions, such as very extensive swelling, redness and severe pain, occur in less than 2% of people who get a booster shot. They are usually adults who have received boosters too often. While pain and tenderness may limit arm movement for a few days, these reactions cause no permanent damage. **Having a large reaction to a previous dose is not a reason to avoid future boosters, if needed.**

- Fever occurs in about 15% of immunized children, but high fever (39°C or higher) and febrile seizures are rare.

- Other side effects in infants may include fussiness, crying, drowsiness, reduced appetite and vomiting. These reactions are usually mild and occur in about half of vaccinated infants. Older children, teens and adults may complain of headache, fatigue and muscle aches.

Rare reactions:
- Severe reactions, such as prolonged inconsolable crying for more than 3 hours, are rare.

- Sudden episodes where an infant becomes limp, less responsive and pale (hypotensive-hyporesponsive events) have been reported, very occasionally, after vaccines containing pertussis. These reactions are rare with today's vaccines but were more common with older forms of pertussis vaccine, which contained whole inactivated bacteria. These reactions are thought to be an infant response to pain, similar to a fainting in an older child or adult, and have no long-term effects.

Measles-mumps-rubella (MMR) and measles-mumps-rubella-varicella (MMRV) vaccines

Side effects after MMR vaccine are usually mild after the first dose and uncommon after the second dose.

Common reactions to MMR:

- **Fever and rash.** The most common side effect is fever. Six to 23 days after receiving MMR vaccine, about 5% of children have fever (with or without a mild rash) lasting for 1 to 3 days. Occasionally, fever is high enough to cause a febrile seizure in children who are susceptible. However, these side effects from *vaccine* are much less severe than the measles *illness*, which causes a more severe and long-lasting rash with fever, red eyes and cough.

- **Other possible side effects.** Occasionally, swollen glands or joint pain may occur after receiving MMR vaccine. Joint pain is rare in children and more common in adolescents or adults. However, adults are three to four times more likely to experience joint pain following rubella *infection* than following MMR *vaccine*.

Common reactions to MMRV:

In addition to the side effects described above with MMR:

- **Injection site reactions.** Pain or soreness, redness, swelling, itching and/or rash at the injection site occur in about 10% to 20% of children after the first dose of vaccine. These reactions are almost always mild and brief.

- **Fever.** A fever of less than 39°C occurs in 20% of children. This reaction is more common than with MMR or chickenpox vaccine alone. Fever over 39°C is also more common than with MMR or chickenpox vaccine alone. Febrile seizures are also slightly more common after a first dose of MMRV than after MMR.

- **Rash.** In addition to the rash described with MMR, a chickenpox-like rash, usually consisting of 10 pox (lesions) or fewer, occurs around the injection site 6 to 23 days after vaccination in less than 5% of children after vaccination.

Rare and more serious reactions to MMR or MMRV:
Serious reactions to MMR or MMRV are *very rare* in healthy children.

- **Meningitis** has been reported to occur at a rate of less than one case per million doses of vaccine, with no permanent brain damage. By comparison, meningitis is very common with mumps infection.

- **Encephalitis** (brain inflammation) occurs in about one case per million doses of vaccine, but it is not known for sure whether the vaccine is responsible. On the other hand, measles *disease* causes encephalitis in about one of every 1000 cases.

- **Thrombocytopenia** (low blood platelets) occurs in a few children (3 or 4 per 100,000 doses of vaccine) within 6 weeks of receiving MMR or MMRV vaccine. The decrease in platelets causes small hemorrhages and bruises in the skin, but serious bleeding is rare. It is probably due to the rubella component of the vaccine and usually resolves within 3 months with no serious complications. Thrombocytopenia is more than 10 times more common after *infection* with rubella than after these vaccines.

- A very few cases of **shingles** (zoster) have been reported after vaccination. These have been mild, with no chronic pain or other complications. The rate of shingles is very much higher after natural chickenpox.

- Measles vaccine is a live vaccine and has caused serious diseases such as encephalitis and severe pneumonia when given inadvertently to a few individuals whose immune system was severely compromised by disease or treatment.

Reasons to delay or avoid a vaccine

When should vaccination be delayed?

- If a child has a **serious illness**, especially when you don't yet know what is wrong (e.g., unexplained fever and not looking well or severe vomiting), a scheduled vaccination should be delayed until the diagnosis is clear or the child has recovered.

> **Not sure whether your child is too sick to be vaccinated?**
>
> Phone ahead and ask your child's doctor or a clinic nurse.

- Infants with **moderate or severe diarrhea** should not receive rotavirus vaccine until they are better, because the vaccine may not work.

- Anyone with **severe nasal congestion** should not receive the live form of influenza vaccine, which is given by nose spray, because the vaccine may not get to the lining of the nose. The inactivated influenza vaccine can be given, or the live vaccine once congestion is gone.

- Anyone who has received an injection of **blood or blood products** (platelets, plasma or immune globulin) should not receive certain live vaccines (measles, mumps, rubella, chickenpox [varicella]) for 3 to 11 months afterward, depending on the amount of blood product injected. These vaccines do not cause any harm if given but the antibodies in blood or blood products can inactivate the vaccine.

- Anyone with **severe asthma** (currently on oral or high-dose inhaled steroids or with active wheezing or wheezing severe enough to have seen a doctor in the past 7 days) should not receive live influenza vaccine, which might cause or aggravate wheezing. The inactivated influenza vaccine can be given. The live vaccine can be given to people whose asthma is stable.

- Someone with active **untreated tuberculosis** (TB) should not receive measles vaccine until treatment for TB has been started.

- Taking **antibiotics** does not interfere with immune response to any routine vaccines. Antibiotics *may* interfere with the action of some live travel vaccines. (For more information, see the Appendix to this book, "Vaccines for foreign travel").

- **Antiviral drugs** active against the chickenpox (varicella) virus, such as acyclovir, valacyclovir and famciclovir, will interfere with the action of chickenpox and shingles (zoster) vaccines. Antivirals against influenza virus (oseltamivir, zanamivir) will prevent the live influenza vaccine from working. For more information, see Chapters 7 and 13, Chickenpox and Influenza.

- Live influenza vaccine and chickenpox vaccine should not be given to children or adolescents who are receiving salicylates **(acetylsalicylic acid, aspirin,** or **ASA)**. This is a precaution: salicylates have been associated with Reye's syndrome, a serious disease of the liver and brain, but only when these drugs were given to children *infected* with influenza or chickenpox. Reye's syndrome has never been reported in connection with these *vaccines*.

- Shingles (zoster) vaccine should be delayed at least one year after having **shingles**.

What conditions *are not* reasons to delay or avoid vaccination?

Vaccination should *not* be delayed because of minor illnesses (such as a cold, cough, ear infection or mild diarrhea) with or without fever, or because a person is taking an antibiotic. Children often have mild illnesses of this sort and delaying vaccination for each episode would have a big impact on optimal timelines for vaccination. Children respond normally to vaccination during these illnesses and have no added side effects.

> ### As a general rule...
> ...anyone who is well enough to go to an appointment for a vaccine is well enough to be immunized.

Having a history of seizures or a neurologic disorder are *not* reasons to avoid vaccines. Many of the infections that vaccines prevent can provoke seizures or make a neurologic condition worse.

Reactions after a previous dose of vaccine that are *not* contraindications to further doses:

- **High fever** (39°C or higher) is common in young children, especially after the first dose of a vaccine. If your child is uncomfortable, you can give acetaminophen or ibuprofen.

- **Febrile seizures** are common and may occur after fever caused by an infection or a vaccine. Most febrile seizures are brief and mild. If your child has had a febrile seizure after a vaccine, ask your doctor what to do if this happens again.

- Vaccines are safe to give when there is a history of **fainting** after a vaccine. Relaxation techniques and being immunized while seated or lying down can help prevent fainting. For more information, see "Minimizing pain and discomfort" in Chapter 4.

- Infants who become limp, pale and less responsive after a vaccine (**hypotonic-hyporesponsive events**) are thought to be reacting to pain and may be vaccinated again, with attention to pain control.

- **Prolonged inconsolable crying** for more than 3 hours after a vaccine is given is probably due to pain at the injection site in babies too young to be able to say they are in pain. Giving acetaminophen or ibuprofen may help.

- Having a **large local reaction** at the injection site (redness or swelling that is bigger than 5 cm or 2 in. in size) after a dose of vaccine *doesn't* mean a person is more likely to have injection site reactions to other vaccines. But another dose of the vaccine that caused the large reaction may cause a similar reaction. Pain relievers such as acetaminophen or ibuprofen sometimes help.

- Severe injection site reactions with **extensive limb swelling** are rare in children but occasionally happen in adults after diphtheria or tetanus vaccines. They may be the result of having doses of these vaccines too close together. An adult who experiences extensive limb swelling should not get another dose of that vaccine for at least 10 years *unless* the vaccine is needed for a tetanus-prone injury.

Who should not be vaccinated?

- Anyone with a **serious disorder of the immune system** should not receive live vaccines: measles, mumps, rubella, chickenpox (varicella) or shingles (zoster), rotavirus, the live form of influenza vaccine, or live vaccines sometimes given for travel. For information, see "Immunocompromising conditions" in Chapter 3.

- Live vaccines (measles, mumps, rubella, chickenpox [varicella], the live form of influenza vaccine, or live vaccines sometimes given for travel) are not given in **pregnancy** because of *theoretical* concern for possible effects on the developing fetus. However, there is *no evidence* that the live vaccines in use today have any harmful effects when given during pregnancy.

- In general, anyone who has had **anaphylaxis after a vaccine** should not be given another dose of that vaccine until the cause of the reaction has been determined. Anaphylaxis is a severe allergic reaction where a person has breathing difficulty and may go into shock due to a drop in blood pressure. The face or lips may also swell. Anaphylaxis usually occurs within minutes of exposure to the source of the allergy. Children who have this type of allergic reaction after a vaccination should be seen and evaluated by a physician to identify the cause. If the vaccine is found to be responsible and the likelihood of being exposed to that infection is very low, the child should not receive another dose of that specific vaccine. If further doses are required because exposure is likely and the child is at risk for serious disease, the vaccine may be given in a special clinic equipped to prevent and control anaphylaxis.

- Allergic reactions to additives in vaccines (e.g., gelatin, neomycin) or to latex (in vaccine containers) are rare, especially in infants. For more information, see "Vaccine additives" in Chapter 4. A person known to have had a **severe allergic reaction to a vaccine additive or to latex** should be assessed by a specialist in allergies before being given that vaccine.

- A form of paralysis called **Guillain-Barré syndrome** (GBS) occurs only rarely after receiving a vaccine but often follows an infection. GBS has been reported after influenza vaccine, at a rate of about one case per million people vaccinated, but influenza *infection* is a much more common cause of GBS. Cases of GBS have been reported after other vaccines, though so rarely it is unclear whether the vaccine was responsible. People who develop GBS within 6 weeks of a vaccine should not have a further dose of that specific vaccine unless another cause was found for their reaction.

- Infants with a history of **intussusception** (a type of bowel obstruction) or with a malformed gastrointestinal tract which has not been corrected by surgery and which could cause intussusception, should not be given the rotavirus vaccine.

- **Thrombocytopenia** (low blood platelets) occurs rarely after measles-mumps-rubella or measles-mumps-rubella-varicella vaccine. It usually resolves within 3 months. If this condition occurs after a first dose of the vaccine, the need to give the second dose should be assessed by a physician.

Vaccine fears

Several disorders have been unjustly linked to vaccines. What these disorders have in common is that their cause is not known. Since most people with these disorders were vaccinated in early childhood, it is easy to blame a vaccine when no other cause can be found. However, there is no evidence to prove that these conditions are caused by vaccination. This section describes some common concerns.

Can measles vaccine or measles-mumps-rubella (MMR) vaccine cause autism or other developmental disorders?

The answer is no. The root of this mistaken idea is a theory proposed by a British physician in 1998, which claimed that immunization with measles, mumps and rubella vaccine caused autism. His original report has since been shown to be fraudulent and was withdrawn by the journal that published it.

Many credible studies were done after his claim was published, all of which found *no* scientific evidence to support his theory:

- A large study of children with autism in England found *no* association between the date at which MMR vaccine was given and the date when parents first became concerned about abnormal behaviour in their child.

- Another study of 463 children with autism born in London between 1979 and 1998 found no change in the proportions of children whose development suddenly regressed after MMR vaccine was introduced in 1988. There were no differences in rates of regression in children who received MMR before their parents became concerned about their development compared with the rates in children who received MMR after the onset of autism or in children who did not receive the vaccine.

- A study of all 537,303 children born in Denmark between 1991 and 1998 found no difference in the rates of autism between children vaccinated with MMR and unvaccinated children.

A Canadian study agreed

A study in Montreal of 27,749 children born between 1987 and 1998 found that the rate of autism increased even when the proportion of children vaccinated with MMR decreased. Moreover, there was no increase in the rate of autism after 1996, when the schedule was changed to two doses of MMR rather than one dose.

- The frequency of autism in the United States and Canada *appears* to have increased in recent years. However, this increase started many years after MMR vaccine was introduced. No increase in autism rates was observed after MMR was first introduced in Canada, the United States, Europe or Japan.

- A separate Swedish study found no difference in the frequency of autism among children born before and after the introduction of MMR vaccine in Sweden.

- In the United Kingdom, autism rates increased almost fourfold in boys who were born between 1988 and 1993, although the MMR vaccination rate was over 95% at the beginning of—and did not change during—this period. Also, the rates of MMR vaccination were the same in children with and without autism.

- In California, between 1980 and 1994, the number of children with autism enrolled in State Developmental Services programs increased by 373%, while the MMR vaccination rate increased by only 14%.

All published and unpublished evidence about MMR vaccine and autism has been reviewed independently by expert committees of the Institute of Medicine in the United States and the American Academy of Pediatrics. Both groups concluded that *there is no scientific evidence to support the theory that MMR causes autism or autistic spectrum disorders.*

Others have expressed concern that giving too many vaccines too soon may cause autism. A study in the United States that compared children who received vaccines according to the routine schedules with those whose vaccines were delayed or who were not vaccinated showed no difference in the frequency of autism.

What, then, could explain the rise in autism rates in some parts of the world?

The most logical explanation is a change in the way the condition is diagnosed. Since 1990, there have been major changes in the criteria used to diagnose autism. Such changes have broadened the scope of the disorder to include many children with milder and atypical forms of autism. There is also much greater public awareness of autism, and more parents are seeking help for their children.

Can pertussis vaccines cause brain damage?

The answer is no. The original pertussis vaccine made from killed whole bacteria caused high fevers and was sometimes blamed for causing brain damage in infants and young children. A review of all of the scientific evidence carried out by the Institute of Medicine in the United States found that there is *no* proof that pertussis vaccine causes brain damage.

By contrast, and based on medical fact, pertussis *infection* can cause seizures, brain damage and infant death. The following facts make it extremely unlikely that pertussis vaccine can cause brain damage:

- Acute illness involving the brain has not been shown to be more common after vaccination than at any other time (except for febrile seizures, which do not cause brain damage).

- Four American studies were carried out involving more than 415,000 children who collectively had received nearly one million doses of pertussis vaccine. The studies failed to find a single case of acute illness involving the brain, other than reports of febrile seizures.

- A study in the United Kingdom was also unable to find a single case of permanent brain damage that was clearly the result of pertussis vaccination. If brain damage does occur after vaccination, it is *extremely* rare.

- When the recommended age for vaccination with pertussis vaccine was lowered in Denmark (from 5 months to 5 weeks) and raised in Japan (from 2 months to 2 years), there was no change in the age of onset of neurologic disease in infants.

- In searching for a link between brain damage and pertussis vaccine, no pattern of symptoms or laboratory test abnormalities have been found and examinations of brains after death found no signs to indicate that pertussis vaccine caused brain trauma. No plausible mechanism has been found by which pertussis vaccination could cause brain damage.

- A study in the United Kingdom found that children who developed infantile spasms (a type of seizure disorder with developmental delay) were *less likely* to have received pertussis vaccine within the last 28 days than children who did *not* develop infantile spasms.

Why then, has pertussis vaccine (along with many other vaccines) been blamed for causing brain damage?

Vaccination is a very common and recognizable event in the first 6 months of most babies' lives. Brain abnormalities, on the other hand, are uncommon and often unrecognizable in the first 6 months of life. Most infants who have malformations of the brain or who suffer brain damage before birth or during labour and delivery appear to be normal for the first few months of life because the brain is not fully developed. Many babies are 4 to 6 months of age or older before it becomes clear that something is wrong with their development.

The diagnosis of cerebral palsy, mental retardation or developmental delay usually cannot be made until an infant is several months old. By then, an infant has already received one or more vaccinations, often with minor side effects such as fever, crying and fussiness. Because this infant appeared to be normal in the first few months of life, the vaccine is blamed. (See Chapter 5 for a discussion of temporal association and cause and effect.)

Can vaccination cause SIDS?

Claims have been made that babies have died of sudden infant death syndrome (SIDS) following vaccination. About 2,500 infants die of SIDS every year in the United States. Since most of these deaths occur before infants are 6 months old, it is to be expected that some of these children had been vaccinated shortly before they died. There is *no* scientific evidence that immunization causes SIDS.

- Several large studies have found no association between vaccination and SIDS.

- In fact, scientific studies in the United States, England and France found that infants who died of SIDS were *less likely* to have been vaccinated recently than infants in the control group (infants in the study who did not die).

- In Sweden, no change in the incidence of SIDS was observed after the discontinuation or decrease of pertussis vaccination in 1979.

- Similarly, in Japan and England, there was no change in the number of SIDS cases when vaccination rates declined in the 1970s.

- In Canada, the United States and other countries, the number of SIDS deaths has decreased markedly in recent years. This decrease in cases is due to the success of the "Back to sleep" campaign, which advises parents to place babies on their backs for sleeping (rather than on their tummies, as was the practice formerly endorsed by paediatricians).

Most cases of SIDS occur in infants younger than 6 months old, the same period during which babies are first vaccinated. Therefore, the probability of vaccination and SIDS occurring within a short time is extremely high. However, the number of deaths after vaccination is no greater than would be expected by chance alone. The association between vaccination and SIDS is purely coincidental.

Can vaccines cause type 1 diabetes?

Type 1 diabetes, formerly known as juvenile or insulin-dependent diabetes, occurs primarily in children, but individuals of all ages can develop the disease. Most cases of type 1 diabetes are caused by an autoimmune process. Autoimmunity is the development of an immune response directed against one or more organs in the body, which can cause damage. In type 1 diabetes, autoimmune reactions destroy the islet cells in the pancreas, which make insulin.

The following scientific observations lead to the conclusion that there is *no* relationship between vaccination and type 1 diabetes:

- The incidence of type 1 diabetes has increased in many countries. However, such increases have not been associated with the introduction of any new childhood vaccines.

- Many studies have shown no increase in type 1 diabetes after vaccination with specific vaccines. Others have shown no differences in vaccination rates of children with type 1 diabetes compared with the vaccination rates of children without diabetes.

- Vaccination rates are the same for children who have antibodies to islet cell antigens and children who do not have such antibodies.

- Studies in mice genetically predisposed to develop type 1 diabetes show no effect of vaccines on the onset of the disorder.

While the cause of type 1 diabetes is not known, there is some evidence to suggest that viral infections may be important triggers for this process in children.

Can vaccines cause asthma and other kinds of allergic disease?

There are certainly many anecdotes claiming that asthma, eczema or some other kind of allergy developed after vaccination. However, recent studies have shown that immunization does not increase the frequency of asthma and other allergic diseases in children.

- A large international study analyzed immunization rates and rates of asthma and other allergic diseases. Researchers obtained rates for 6- and 7-year-olds from 91 centres in 38 countries, and for 13- and 14-year-olds from 99 centres in 41 countries. They found *no* correlation between immunization rates and asthma or allergy rates.

- A study of 1,366 infants with wheezing showed no relation with vaccination.

- In a study of 165,000 children, childhood vaccinations were not associated with increased risk for asthma.

Can vaccination cause cancer?

While cancer is relatively uncommon in children, affecting about 1 in 10,000 children under 15 years old, it is now the second most common cause of death in children (injuries being number one). There has been no significant increase in leukemia or other cancers in children since the start of routine vaccination in the 1940s. While it is difficult to prove that immunization never causes cancer, there is no scientific evidence of a link between the two.

However, vaccines can *prevent* some types of cancer. People infected with hepatitis B virus are over 40 times more likely to develop cancer of the liver than people not infected. The vaccine prevents infection with hepatitis B virus and this, in turn, prevents the liver cancer. Routine immunization of all infants in Taiwan has been shown to prevent both infection with hepatitis B and liver cancer caused by hepatitis B. Similarly, the human papillomavirus vaccine prevents the most common sexually transmitted disease in Canada as well cervical cancer later in life.

Can vaccines cause Crohn's disease or ulcerative colitis?

It has been claimed that Crohn's disease (a chronic inflammation of the intestines from unknown causes) was more common in young adults who had received measles vaccine than in unvaccinated adults. The same researcher also claimed to have found genetic material of measles virus in samples of intestinal tissue from patients with Crohn's disease.

Additional studies have failed to find *any* association between measles vaccination and Crohn's disease or any other form of inflammatory bowel disease. Moreover, two other laboratories failed to confirm the claim that measles virus is present in samples of inflamed tissue from patients with Crohn's disease.

Can vaccines cause multiple sclerosis?

There are more cases of multiple sclerosis (MS) today than 30 or more years ago. The reasons for this increase are earlier and improved methods of diagnosis, improved treatment and longer survival of MS patients. The cause of MS is not yet known.

There is some evidence suggesting that infection in childhood might play a role in the development of this disease. There is no evidence that immunization causes MS or even flare-ups in a person with MS. In particular, hepatitis B and influenza vaccines have been shown to have no effect on symptoms or on the rate that symptoms progress in patients with MS. By contrast, influenza *infection* has been associated with flare-ups of MS.

Can vaccines cause chronic fatigue syndrome?

The cause of chronic fatigue syndrome is not known. Some opponents of vaccination have alleged that hepatitis B vaccination causes this illness. However, studies comparing vaccinated and unvaccinated adults did not show any increased risk of chronic fatigue syndrome after vaccination.

Benefits and risks: Comparing effects of diseases and vaccines

The risks associated with the vaccines that are routinely given to children in Canada are much, much less than the risks associated with the diseases themselves . The following section highlights the effects of these diseases and of the vaccines that protect against them. The information on benefits and risks is summarized in Table 6.1.

Chickenpox is a mild disease in most children, but complications occur in 5% to 10% of previously healthy children. Complications include severe skin infections, pneumonia, encephalitis and cerebellar ataxia, some of which can lead to death. Even uncomplicated chickenpox cases come with a high price tag: costs of visits to doctors and medications; days lost from child care or school; and the time and salary lost by parents who stay home to care for sick children. Chickenpox is a much more severe disease in adolescents and adults, who have higher rates of complications and death from chickenpox than younger age groups.

Chickenpox vaccine may occasionally cause a few skin lesions, especially around the injection site, but not the complications of chickenpox.

Diphtheria and tetanus can be fatal. Diphtheria kills 1 in every 10 persons who get the illness. Tetanus kills from 10% to 80% of people who become infected, with highest rates in infants and elderly people.

Serious reactions after both vaccines are extremely rare.

Hib, meningococcus and **pneumococcus** bacteria cause meningitis and other life-threatening infections, such as bacteremia (blood infection) and pneumonia. Even with treatment, 5% to 20% of children with meningitis die and a similar proportion of survivors have deafness or brain damage.

The Hib, meningococcal and pneumococcal vaccines are extremely safe, with serious reactions happening very rarely, if at all.

Hepatitis A infects the liver and causes hepatitis. Many children infected with hepatitis A do not get sick or just have a fever. However, children with no symptoms are still contagious and can spread the virus to others. People who do get sick have fever, fatigue, loss of appetite, nausea, vomiting, and yellow skin and eyes (jaundice). Recovery usually takes weeks. Sometimes, though rarely, the infection is so severe that it causes death.

The hepatitis A vaccine is safe. Serious reactions are very rare, if they occur at all.

Hepatitis B virus also infects the liver. Young children often don't get sick at the time. Older children and adults may have fever, fatigue, loss of appetite, nausea, vomiting, and yellow skin and eyes (jaundice). Children often develop a chronic infection, which eventually leads to liver failure or cancer when they become adults.

The hepatitis B vaccine is very effective and has no proven serious side effects.

Human papillomavirus (HPV) infections are very common. About 3 out of 4 sexually active Canadians will be infected with HPV during their lifetime. Some strains of HPV cause cervical cancer. About 1,300 Canadian women are diagnosed with cervical cancer and about 350 women die each year of the disease. HPV also causes cancer of the vulva or vagina in women and cancer of the penis in men. Other strains of HPV cause common warts and genital warts.

Serious side effects after HPV vaccine are rare and not necessarily related to the vaccine.

Measles causes encephalitis (brain inflammation) in about one of every 1,000 cases. One-third of people with measles encephalitis die, and one-third survive with brain damage.

Encephalitis has been reported in about one case per million doses of measles vaccine. This occurrence rate is so low that it is unclear whether the vaccine is even responsible.

Mumps meningitis occurs in about 5% of mumps cases and infection with mumps virus causes deafness in 0.5 to 5 out of every 100,000 cases.

Meningitis is reported to occur at a rate of less than one case per million doses of vaccine and has no long-term complications.

Pertussis kills 1 to 4 infants every year in Canada, and about 1 in 400 hospitalized with the disease dies of either pneumonia or brain damage.

There is no evidence that pertussis vaccine causes brain damage.

Rotavirus causes very profuse, watery diarrhea and vomiting that can rapidly lead to dehydration. Before we had the vaccine, almost 1% of children were hospitalized with rotavirus before their 5th birthday.

Rotavirus vaccine is very safe. In very rare cases (about 1 to 5 children in 100,000), vaccination may be followed by a type of bowel obstruction called intussusception. This condition also occurs after rotavirus infection.

Rubella infection during the first 20 weeks of pregnancy means chances are high (more than 8 in 10) that the fetus will be infected. Infection of the fetus can cause heart abnormalities, deafness, blindness and severe learning problems.

Rubella vaccine sometimes causes joint pain in adult women. But joint pain is more common and more severe after rubella infection than after vaccine.

Table 6.1
Summary of effects of diseases and corresponding vaccines

Disease	Average number of cases and related deaths each year in Canada		Effects of disease	Side effects of vaccine
	Before vaccine available*	After vaccine available*		
Chickenpox	350,000 cases, 1500–2000 hospitalizations, 10 deaths	80% decrease in hospitalization of children	Complications in 5% to 10% of previously healthy children, e.g., severe skin infections, flesh-eating disease, pneumonia. Encephalitis in 1 per 5,000 cases. Birth deformities in 1% to 2% of infants of mothers with chickenpox in first 20 weeks of pregnancy. Shingles (zoster) later in life.	Mild pain, redness at injection site in 10% to 20% of recipients. Fever <39°C in 10% to 15%. Chickenpox-like rash at injection site (day 6–23) in 3% to 5%. (For measles-mumps-rubella-varicella vaccine, see Measles, below.)
Diphtheria	12,000 cases with 1,000 deaths	0–5 cases with 0 deaths	Severe sore throat, severe breathing difficulty, suffocation, marked weakness, nerve damage, heart failure. Death in 5% to 10% of cases.	Combined vaccine: diphtheria-tetanus-pertussis-polio-Hib. 10% to 40% of infants have mild redness, swelling and pain at the injection site; larger reactions with booster at 4 to 6 yrs old. Mild fever in 15%.

* In the past 6 to 10 years

Disease	Average number of cases and related deaths each year in Canada		Effects of disease	Side effects of vaccine
	Before vaccine available*	After vaccine available*		
Haeemophilus influenzae type b	1,500 cases of meningitis and 1,500 cases of infections of blood, bone, lungs, skin, joints (1 child in 300 infected)	About 30 cases	Meningitis kills in 5% of cases, leads to brain damage in 10% to 15% and deafness in 15% to 20% of survivors.	See Diphtheria, above.
Hepatitis A	10–20,000 cases	>90% decrease in cases	25% of adults are hospitalized. Death from overwhelming liver damage in a very small proportion of cases.	Mild pain and redness at injection site.
Hepatitis B	20,000 new cases per year with 480–500 deaths	<1,000 cases, decreased by >90%	90% of infants and 10% of adults develop chronic disease. Death in 25% from complications of chronic infection (i.e., cirrhosis, liver cancer). Severe acute illness may also cause death.	Mild pain and redness at injection site in 10% to 15% of recipients.
Human papillomavirus	Affects 75% of sexually active Canadians. 1,300 cases of cervical cancer, with 350 deaths.	Too new to see effect.	Cancer of cervix, vagina, vulva. Cancer of anus, penis. Genital and anal warts.	Mild pain and redness at injection site.
Influenza	Immunity short-term only; I0% to 20% of population infected each year, with an estimated 12,000 hospitalizations and 3,500 deaths. Young children, people with chronic diseases and the elderly more often hospitalized. Those with chronic diseases and the elderly are more likely to die. Annual immunization of high-risk people reduced hospitalization rates by 50% to 70% and deaths in the elderly by about 85%.		High fever, febrile convulsions in young children; pneumonia, muscle inflammation. Rarely, inflammation of the brain or heart.	Injectable vaccine: • Mild pain at injection site. • Mild fever in up to 12% of children. • Very rarely, Guillain-Barré syndrome, a form of muscle paralysis (1 per million doses). Intranasal vaccine: • Mild nasal congestion and runny nose.

* In the past 6 to 10 years

Disease	Average number of cases and related deaths each year in Canada		Effects of disease	Side effects of vaccine
	Before vaccine available*	After vaccine available*		
Measles	95% of children had measles by age 18. 300,000 cases with 300 deaths and 400 children with brain damage.	60–750 cases	Severe bronchitis, high fever, rash for 7–14 days. Pneumonia in 1 in 10 cases. Encephalitis in 1 in 1,000 cases; 15% with encephalitis die and 25% have permanent brain damage. Death in 1–2 per 1,000 cases.	Combined vaccines: Measles-mumps-rubella-chickenpox vaccine • 5% of recipients have fever with or without a mild rash 6–23 days after vaccine. • Swollen glands in a few cases. • Joint pain in adolescent or adult women (1 in 7). • Febrile seizures in about 1 per 2,500–4,000 doses. • Low platelets in 1 per 25,000 doses. • Encephalitis in 1 per one million doses. Measles-mumps-rubella-chickenpox vaccine • Fever <39°C in 20% of recipients. • Chickenpox-like rash at injection site (day 6–23) in 3% to 5%. • Febrile seizures more common than with measles-mumps-rubella vaccine (1 in 1,250-2,500 with first dose).
Meningococcus group C	Group C: 186	Group C: 29 (B is now the most common in Canada.)	Death in 10% of cases; brain damage, deafness, amputations, skin loss in 10% to 20% of survivors.	Mild redness, swelling and pain at the injection site in 10% to 50% of recipients.
Mumps	34,000 cases	200–1000 cases	Fever, swollen salivary glands. Meningitis in 5% of cases; occasional infertility in males. Encephalitis in 1 per 50,000; deafness in 0.5 to 5 per 100,000 cases.	See Measles and Chickenpox, above.

* In the past 6 to 10 years

Disease	Average number of cases and related deaths each year in Canada		Effects of disease	Side effects of vaccine
	Before vaccine available*	After vaccine available*		
Pertussis	30,000–50,000 cases with 50–100 deaths	700–4000 cases with 1–4 deaths	Severe coughing spasms lasting 3–6 weeks, pneumonia, convulsions. Death from brain damage or pneumonia in 1 of every 400 hospitalized infants.	See Diphtheria, above. There is no evidence that pertussis vaccine causes brain damage.
Pneumococcus	3,000 cases of severe disease (meningitis, bacteremia, pneumonia) in children <5 yrs old	275–375 cases <5 yrs old; decrease of 79% in children <2 yrs old	Death in approximately 10% of cases with meningitis; 10% to 15% of survivors of meningitis have brain damage, 5% to 10% have deafness. Death in 5% to 7% of cases with pneumonia.	Mild redness, swelling and pain at injection site in 15% of recipients.
Polio	2,000 cases in last epidemic in 1959	0 (last case in 1989)	Muscle paralysis in 1 out of 100 persons infected with polio. Death in 2% to 5% of children and 15% to 30% of adults with paralytic disease.	See Diphtheria, above.
Rotavirus	400,000 cases; 1% of children hospitalized by age 5 yrs. 2–4 deaths in children <2 yrs old.	Too new to see effect.	Death from severe dehydration caused by profuse, watery diarrhea.	Very rare cases of bowel obstruction (intussusception): 1–5 in 100,000 doses.
Rubella	85% of children had rubella by age 20, or 250,000 cases. About 200 cases of congenital rubella syndrome.	2–13 cases. 0–1 babies with congenital rubella syndrome born to unvaccinated mothers.	Fever, swollen glands, rash. Joint pain, arthritis in adults. Severe damage to fetus if mother infected during first trimester of pregnancy.	See Measles and Chickenpox, above.
Tetanus	60–75 cases, with 40–50 deaths.	1–6 cases	Toxin affects spinal cord, leading to painful muscle spasms and seizures. Death in 10% to 80% of cases.	See Diphtheria, above.

* In the past 6 to 10 years

II

Vaccine-preventable diseases

7

Chickenpox and shingles

Chickenpox (also known as varicella) is a very contagious infection caused by the varicella-zoster (VZ) virus. VZ virus also causes zoster, usually called "shingles". People get chickenpox after their first infection with VZ virus. Shingles can occur years or even decades after the first infection.

Chickenpox commonly causes fever, headache, aches and pains, and a very itchy rash. It can lead to complications requiring hospitalization and, in rare cases, to death. Most cases are in children younger than 15 years old. The illness is more severe in teenagers and adults than in children.

First infections with the virus are known as chickenpox, regardless of the age at which a person becomes infected.

Shingles is caused by reactivation of the VZ virus, which stays in certain nerve cells in a latent (inactive) form after chickenpox infection. A localized rash, usually very itchy and painful, is the main symptom of shingles, and chronic pain at the site of the rash is its main complication.

The vaccine against chickenpox is often called "varicella vaccine", while the vaccine against shingles is often called "zoster vaccine".

A history of chickenpox

Before vaccine

About 95% of Canadians used to be infected with VZ virus during their lifetime, with over 300,000 cases of chickenpox occurring each year. More than 90% of cases were in children younger than 15 years of age, with the highest rates in 5- to 9-year-olds. While many cases were mild, especially in young children, there were also 1,500 to 2,000 hospitalizations and an average of 10 deaths each year. The death rate in children was 1 to 3 per 100,000 cases.

After vaccine

The chickenpox vaccine was approved for use in Canada in 1998 and has been included in routine childhood vaccination programs since 2006. A two-dose schedule for all children was recommended in 2010.

The number of children hospitalized with chickenpox began to drop dramatically as soon as these programs began. Between 2000–01 and 2008, the yearly average number of hospitalizations for chickenpox in the 12 leading paediatric hospitals had dropped by over 80%. Since 2000, IMPACT has reported 11 paediatric deaths from chickenpox, with between 0 and 3 deaths per year.

In the United States, the chickenpox vaccine has been available since 1995. Many states now require proof of vaccination against chickenpox before children can attend school. In the early 1990s, an average of 4 million people in the United States got chickenpox, 10,500 to 13,000 were hospitalized, and 100 to 150 died each year. Today, more than 3.5 million cases of chickenpox, along with 9,000 hospitalizations and 100 deaths, are being prevented each year by the chickenpox vaccine in the United States!

More reasons to immunize

Although most cases of chickenpox are mild to moderate, potential complications of chickenpox, such as pneumonia, encephalitis and cerebellar ataxia, can be severe and even lead to death.

People with chickenpox usually have between 250 and 500 "pox", an extremely itchy rash that can be very uncomfortable.

Apart from the health-risk factors, there is a high price tag associated with chickenpox, even for uncomplicated cases: the costs of doctor visits, medications, days lost from school or paid child care, and the time and salary lost by parents who stay home to care for a sick child. One Canadian study showed that between 30% and 65% of children with chickenpox were seen by a doctor.

A recently redeveloped **shingles vaccine** is very effective in preventing shingles among older adults.

The germ

Varicella-zoster (VZ) virus is a member of the herpes family of viruses, which also includes the virus that causes cold sores. When illness is gone, herpes viruses stay in the body, causing a latent (or silent) infection that lasts for life. VZ virus only infects humans.

After the **first infection as chickenpox**, VZ virus infects specialized nerve cells of the dorsal root ganglia, which are next to the spinal cord. During this latent phase of infection, there are no symptoms or other evidence that VZ virus is in the body.

Reinfection(s). A new, second infection with VZ virus can happen but in most cases produces no illness and can be detected only by special laboratory tests. Only rarely does a reinfection result in a second attack of chickenpox.

Reactivation as shingles. Immunity to chickenpox develops after infection, which lowers the risk of illness when a person is exposed to chickenpox again. But this immune response cannot get rid of the VZ virus, which stays in the body for life. In some people, usually adults, the virus starts to grow again, spreading down the nerve fibres to the skin. About 10% to 15% of people infected with VZ virus develop shingles at some time during their lives.

How the germ causes illness

Chickenpox. When someone breathes in droplets containing chicken-pox virus, the virus first infects cells lining the nose and throat. It then spreads to lymph glands in the neck. After multiplying there for a few days, the virus enters the bloodstream and is carried throughout the body to other lymph glands, the liver, spleen and bone marrow, where it grows for another few days. The virus then reinvades the blood and spreads to the skin, eyes, respiratory tract and other organs.

The amount of virus in the blood reaches a peak about 11 to 14 days after exposure, then declines rapidly over the next few days. The second phase of **viremia** (meaning virus present in the blood) coincides with the appearance of fever and the chickenpox rash.

Shingles. The VZ virus reactivates and spreads to the skin. The rash is similar to that of chickenpox, but is localized to the area of skin supplied

---

Young people can also get shingles

Sometimes, healthy children and teens get shingles. This is more likely to happen when a child has a very mild chickenpox infection early in life, so does not develop a solid immune response to the VZ virus.

---

by the nerves that contain infected cells. The risk of developing shingles increases as the interval after having chickenpox gets longer, making the elderly especially vulnerable.

Reactivation is believed to occur as a result of waning immunity to VZ virus because of aging or weakening immune function (i.e., caused by disease, such as cancer, or by a treatment that suppresses the immune system, such as chemotherapy or high-dose steroids).

How VZ virus spreads

Chickenpox spreads very easily from person to person, usually by contact with respiratory secretions or by breathing in airborne droplets containing many virus particles. The skin lesions (pox) can also release virus particles into the air. The virus can survive in the air for several hours. When someone breathes in these particles, cells in the nose and throat become infected.

Highly contagious, easily spread

In a household, chickenpox will spread to 60% to 85% of people who are not already immune to it. The rate of spread of chickenpox is higher in home settings than in child care centres or schools.

Chickenpox cases occur throughout the year but they increase in September, after school opens, peak in the spring, and drop sharply during the summer.

Children are contagious for 1 to 2 days *before* the rash appears. This helps explain the ease of spread. Contagiousness decreases after the rash starts. Children are considered contagious for a minimum of 5 days after the rash appears and until all the pox have crusted. Current CPS policy states that children with mild chickenpox can return to their school or child care program as soon as they feel well enough to participate normally in all activities, regardless of what their rash looks like. The main reason is that by the time the rash appears, spread has likely already happened.

People with **shingles** are also contagious, but only to persons who have never had chickenpox. Virus released from the shingles lesions can also spread through the air. Individuals who are not immune will get chickenpox, not shingles.

Be sure to tell the teacher!

Teachers or child care staff need to be told when a child has chickenpox, so that parents can be notified. All parents should be notified that chickenpox is in a child care program or classroom. Notification is especially important for parents of a child whose immune function is weakened by a chronic illness or ongoing therapy.

Chickenpox: The illness

Symptoms in children (pre-rash). Following an incubation period of 10 to 21 days (average is 14 to 16 days), some children experience a short period (1 to 2 days) of fever (39–40°C) with aches and pains. They may also lose their appetite and have a headache in the first few days of illness. These symptoms are usually not severe.

Rash. In many children, the first sign of illness is the rash. It first appears on the scalp and face and spreads quickly down the body and onto the arms and legs. The rash is more intense on the face and body than on the hands or feet.

Each skin lesion (or pox) moves rapidly through four stages:
• red spot,
• vesicle (a small blister filled with clear fluid),
• pustule (a blister filled with cloudy fluid), then
• crust or scab.

New pox appear in crops for up to 3 to 4 days so that lesions in all stages may be present at the same time. The rash is usually very itchy and uncomfortable.

Symptoms in adolescents and adults are more severe than in children. There are more pox, the fever is higher and the illness lasts longer.

Complications

In children. Complications occur in 5% to 10% of previously healthy children with chickenpox. The most common complications are:
- **bacterial skin infections**
- **pneumonia:** a lung infection
- **encephalitis:** intense inflammation of the brain (1 in 5,000 cases)
- **cerebellar ataxia:** inflammation of a part of the brain called the cerebellum (1 in 4,000 cases). A child with cerebellar ataxia has sudden difficulty with walking, sitting, and other muscle movement.

Flesh-eating disease. More than half of the complications of chickenpox are skin infections caused by scratching an itchy rash. While most skin infections are mild, chickenpox is one of the most common reasons why children get the life-threatening infection called necrotizing fasciitis (or "flesh-eating disease") caused by group A *Streptococcus*. These bacteria can invade the body though the open pox.

Other bacterial infections that can complicate chickenpox are less common but include bacteremia (blood infection), osteomyelitis (bone infection), joint infections and conjunctivitis (inflammation of the eye).

Reye's syndrome, a condition that damages the brain and liver, was more common when children with chickenpox were treated with aspirin. This disorder became very rare after it was recommended *not* to give aspirin to children with fever. Acetaminophen (Tylenol, Tempra) may be given.

In adults. Complications from chickenpox are more frequent and severe in adults. The death rate from chickenpox is about 25 times higher in adults than in children. While only 5% of all chickenpox cases are in adults, 55% to 60% of deaths due to chickenpox are in adults and usually caused by encephalitis or pneumonia (see Table 7.1).

Table 7.1
Complications of chickenpox, by group affected

Complication	Group affected
Bacterial infection of pox	Children
Flesh-eating disease	
Bacteremia, bone and joint infections	
Cerebellar ataxia	
Pneumonia	Adults much more often than children
Encephalitis	
Death	

During pregnancy. If a woman gets chickenpox during her first 20 weeks of pregnancy, there is a risk that the virus will infect the fetus. Called **congenital varicella syndrome**, this infection can cause serious problems (see Table 7.2).

Table 7.2
Congenital varicella syndrome

Feature	Frequency (%)
Severe skin scars	70
Blindness or damaged eyes	66
Low birth weight	50
Abnormal growth of extremities (deformed limbs)	50
Brain damage	45
Death before 14 months of age	28

The risk of congenital varicella syndrome varies, depending on when the mother gets chickenpox:
* In the first trimester (0 to 12 weeks of pregnancy), the risk is 0.4% (4 per 1,000),
* In the second trimester (13 to 20 weeks), the risk increases to 2.0% (20 per 1,000).

The syndrome is very rare when infection occurs after the 20th week of pregnancy.

However, if the mother develops chickenpox around the time of delivery (from 5 days before to 2 days after her baby's birth), up to 30% (3 out of

10) of newborn infants will develop very severe chickenpox, with problems in the brain, heart and liver. If not treated, about 1 in 5 infected newborns will die.

In immunocompromised people. Before current therapies became available, such as specific immune globulin to prevent chickenpox and medications to treat the illness, children with weakened immune function were at high risk for severe chickenpox and often died from the infection. Children with leukemia, lymphoma, a bone marrow or organ transplant, or on a medication that suppressed immune system function, were included in this high-risk group. With current treatments, however, death is now rare in such children.

Diagnosis

The chickenpox rash can usually be diagnosed without laboratory tests, but tests to find the virus in skin lesions or antibodies in blood are available.

Treatment

Antiviral medication

Chickenpox can be treated with a variety of antiviral medications, including acyclovir, valacyclovir and famciclovir, given either by mouth or intravenously (through an intravenous drip administered in the hospital).

Treating otherwise healthy children. Antiviral treatment is *not* routinely used for otherwise healthy children with chickenpox, unless their infection is severe.

Treating people at higher risk for serious disease. Antiviral medications are used to treat the following groups:
- Newborns infected before or during delivery
- Individuals who have a chronic condition or are undergoing treatment that weakens (compromises) immune function, including those receiving corticosteroids
- People with chronic skin or lung disorders

- Children and adolescents on long-term aspirin therapy
- Otherwise healthy adolescents and adults.

Antiviral treatment should be started early because the VZ virus stops multiplying within 72 hours of the rash first appearing in children who have a normal immune response. If possible, treatment should be started within 24 hours of the rash first appearing.

Post-recovery

After infection, antibodies persist for many decades, often for life, but cellular immunity weakens with age, allowing reactivation of latent virus and resulting in shingles.

The vaccine

Type of vaccine

Live attenuated virus vaccine. Chickenpox vaccine is a live virus that has been attenuated (weakened). The vaccine virus multiplies in the body after it is injected but does not cause chickenpox. Instead it imitates natural infection: the virus infects, multiplies and stimulates immunity. The vaccine virus does not cause any illness in most people. See "Possible side effects of chickenpox vaccine", below.

How chickenpox vaccine is made

Producing a weakened strain. Dr. Michiaki Takahashi developed chickenpox vaccine in Japan from a strain of virus isolated from a 3-year-old boy with chickenpox, named K. Oka. The "Oka strain" was weakened by repeatedly growing it human tissue culture cells and guinea pig cells.

Process. The current vaccine is derived from the Oka strain and is produced in human tissue culture cells, called MRC-5 cells. The virus is grown in cell cultures, then extracted, purified and freeze-dried.

For general information on vaccine additives, see Chapter 4.

Available forms of chickenpox vaccine

Alone or in combination. In Canada, chickenpox vaccine is available both as a single vaccine and in combination with measles, mumps and rubella vaccines (known as MMRV).

Vaccine for children, adolescents and adults. The same "chickenpox-only" vaccine is used in children of all ages and in non-immune adults. MMRV, the combination vaccine, isn't given to people over 12 years of age because it has not yet been tested in older age groups.

How the vaccine is given

The freeze-dried vaccine is mixed with sterile distilled water and given as a single injection beneath the skin. The MMRV vaccine may also be injected into muscle. For more information, see "Getting the shot" in Chapter 4.

Schedule of vaccination

Infants and children (under 13 years old). Chickenpox vaccine is given after the first birthday. Children 1 to 12 years old receive 2 doses. The first dose of chickenpox vaccine is given at 12 to 15 months of age. The second dose is given at age 18 months in some provinces or territories and later in others. The second dose must be given, at the latest, before school entry (at 4 to 6 years of age). The optimal age for receiving these doses is being assessed.

Chickenpox vaccine may be given a single vaccine or in combination with others as MMRV.

Before 2011, only one dose of vaccine was recommended for this age group. Today, children who received one dose of the vaccine should get a second dose unless they have had chickenpox since their first dose. However, not all provinces or territories in Canada are providing 2 doses of chickenpox vaccine at this time.

For children who have not been vaccinated according to the routine schedules, the 2 doses of chickenpox vaccine should be *at least* 6 weeks

—and *preferably* 3 months—apart. If MMR and chickenpox vaccine are not given at the same time, they should be given *at least* 4 weeks apart.

Adolescents (13 to 19 years) and adults who have not had chickenpox should receive 2 doses of chickenpox vaccine, given *at least* 6 weeks apart.

Boosters (to enhance prior vaccinations). Currently, boosters of regular chickenpox vaccine are not recommended.

How long the vaccine protects against chickenpox is not yet known, but it is expected to be at least 15 years.

Preventing chickenpox after exposure: Post-exposure control

Vaccine

Chickenpox vaccine may also be given to prevent infection in non-immune individuals who have been exposed to chickenpox. It is effective when it is given within 5 days of first contact with a person with chickenpox or shingles. Vaccination within this time period will either prevent illness altogether or significantly reduce the severity of illness.

Passive immunization: Immune globulin

Non-immune individuals who are at high risk of severe disease (see the text box, below) need protection following exposure to chickenpox. They get a special preparation of immune globulin known as **varicella-zoster immune globulin (VariZIG)**. VariZIG contains a high concentration of antibody against varicella-zoster virus. The antibodies coat the virus particles, enabling white blood cells to destroy the virus before it can cause any damage.

> **After exposure to chickenpox**
> Some non-immune people at high risk of severe disease may be given an injection of antibodies to help protect them until they are able to make their own antibodies. This is known as **passive immunization**.

Does VariZIG work? For best effect, VariZIG should be given as soon as possible after exposure to chickenpox and, ideally, within 96 hours. It can be given later but the benefit is unknown. It is probably most effective when given early after exposure.

How is VariZIG made? VariZIG is prepared from the plasma (the liquid part of blood) of volunteer donors, using methods that concentrate the antibodies. When injected, the recipient gets a concentrated dose of VZ antibody.

Is VariZIG safe? Current methods of testing blood from volunteer donors and of preparing IG ensure that there is no risk of acquiring HIV, hepatitis B, hepatitis C or any other known virus from this product. Other than pain at the injection site, there are almost no significant reactions to IG. Rarely, allergic reactions have been reported.

Who should receive VariZIG after being exposed to chickenpox?

- Non-immune **immunocompromised** people (including those with HIV infection, if they have severe immune deficiency)
- Non-immune **pregnant women**
- **Newborns** whose mothers develop chickenpox from 5 days before to 2 days after delivery
- Hospitalized **premature newborns** whose gestational age is 28 weeks or more, and whose mothers have no history of chickenpox
- Hospitalized **premature newborns** whose gestational age is less than 28 weeks or whose birth weight is less than 1000 g, regardless of their mothers' history of chickenpox

---

Possible side effects of chickenpox vaccine

Giving chickenpox vaccine at the same time as another vaccine does not increase the side effects of either.

Local reactions. Chickenpox vaccine is very safe. Reactions are usually mild. Pain or tenderness, redness, swelling or itching at the injection site occur in about 10% to 20% of children after a single dose of vaccine. These local reactions are almost always mild and brief.

A chickenpox-like rash, usually consisting of no more than 10 pox (lesions) or fewer, occurs around the injection site in less than 5% of children after vaccination.

Fever. A fever of less than 39°C occurs in 10% to 15% of children after chickenpox vaccination (compared with 67% in children who are infected with chickenpox). Fever is more common after receiving MMRV vaccine (at 20%) than after receiving MMR or chickenpox vaccine alone.

There is no evidence that chickenpox vaccine causes serious adverse events.

Transmission of the vaccine virus from healthy vaccinated children to someone who is non-immune has happened, but only in a handful of documented cases. Spread of the vaccine virus from children who have leukemia to non-immune contacts has been more common, but only if these children develop a rash after receiving the VZ vaccine.

Shingles after vaccination can happen, though this too is rare. The rate of shingles is 4 to 12 times lower with the vaccine than following natural chickenpox. Shingles in vaccinated children and adults has been mild, with no chronic pain or other complications observed.

For information on possible reactions after receiving the combined vaccine, see Chapter 6, Adverse events and common concerns.

Reasons to delay or avoid chickenpox vaccine

Immunosuppression (compromised immune function). As with all live virus vaccines, chickenpox vaccine is not usually given to people with a serious immune system disorder caused by disease or certain medications. However, it is sometimes used in circumstances where benefits of receiving the vaccine clearly outweigh the risks. Your doctor or a specialist will discuss your child's particular issues with you if such circumstances arise. For more information, see Chapter 3, When extra protection is needed.

During pregnancy. Chickenpox vaccine is not given in pregnancy because of a *theoretical* risk of transmitting the vaccine virus to the fetus. But there is *no evidence that chickenpox vaccine can harm the fetus*. Ideally, a woman who needs to be immunized should delay pregnancy by 4 weeks following chickenpox vaccination. But if the vaccine was given before she knew she was pregnant, there is no need for concern or for the pregnancy to be terminated. A pregnant women's other children should be vaccinated according to the routine schedule.

Recent injection with IG or other blood products. Immune globulin (IG) and other blood products may contain antibody to varicella virus that will make the chickenpox vaccine inactive. Vaccination must be delayed for 3 to 11 months, depending on the type and dosage of IG or other blood product used.

Antiviral therapy: Antiviral drugs active against varicella virus, specifically acyclovir, valacyclovir and famciclovir, make the chickenpox vaccine inactive. These drugs should not be taken one day before or up to 14 days after chickenpox vaccine has been given.

Aspirin therapy: Chickenpox vaccine should be used with caution in children receiving aspirin or other salicylate therapy (see "Salicylate therapy" in Chapter 3).

For general information on reasons to delay or avoid a vaccine or vaccines, see Chapter 6.

The results of vaccination

Chickenpox vaccine stimulates antibody in over 97% of healthy children after one dose and in adolescents and adults after two doses. But some children apparently lose antibodies over time, especially if they have received only one dose of vaccine, and may become susceptible to chickenpox.

The current vaccine is 85% to 90% effective in preventing chickenpox. Children who get chickenpox despite being vaccinated have a mild illness compared with children who have not been vaccinated. They usually have fewer than 30 pox (compared with the more than 300 typically experienced by an unvaccinated child), a lower occurrence of fever, and a more rapid recovery.

Evidence that chickenpox vaccine works:
- In Canada, the number of children hospitalized because of chickenpox has dropped by over 80% since the vaccine became available. There has also been a 78% decrease in hospitalizations of children younger than 1 year of age (and therefore too young to be vaccinated themselves). They were protected from chickenpox indirectly, because there are fewer infectious older children around.
- In the United States, the reported rate of chickenpox has declined by more than 50%, and the number of related deaths in children by 78%, since the vaccine was introduced.
- Controlled studies have shown that the vaccine reduces the likelihood of getting chickenpox following exposure to an infected family member by over 97%.
- Chickenpox in vaccinated children is much milder than that in unvaccinated children.
- Follow-up of children years after vaccination has shown that protection against chickenpox following exposure to a case lasts at least 7 to 10 years.

Shingles (zoster): The illness

Symptoms. A rash develops on an area of skin on one side of the body. Sometimes there is pain, itching or burning before the rash appears. The rash is similar to chickenpox, except it stays in one area. The rash is almost always very itchy and is often very painful. Without treatment, it lasts 10 to 15 days.

Complications

The most common complication of shingles is a condition called **postherpetic neuralgia**, where constant or intermittent pain occurs in the area of skin affected by shingles after the rash has disappeared. The pain, which can be severe and incapacitating, may last 3 months or more. Although uncommon after shingles in children or young adults, this condition occurs in over 25% of individuals who get shingles after age 50.

In a few people, the shingles rash spreads over the entire body.

If rash is on the eyelids, the cornea can be infected, leading to scarring and possible blindness.

In people with depressed immunity, zoster can cause brain or lung infection.

Diagnosis

The shingles rash is very characteristic and can usually be diagnosed without laboratory tests. The virus can be detected in specimens taken from the skin lesions.

Treatment

Shingles can be treated with a variety of antiviral medications, including acyclovir, valacyclovir and famciclovir, either by mouth or intravenously (through an intravenous drip administered in hospital).

Antiviral drugs can shorten the duration of the shingles rash if they are started within the first 5 days after onset of the rash. These drugs are not of any benefit in treating postherpetic neuralgia. Antiviral treatment is given to all individuals with a disease or undergoing a treatment that compromises immune function.

The vaccine

The shingles vaccine is used as a booster in older adults who have previously had chickenpox and may have a weakening immunity because of their age.

Type of vaccine

Live, attenuated virus vaccine. Shingles (zoster) vaccine is a live virus that has been attenuated (weakened) (see Chickenpox vaccine, above).

How shingles vaccine is made

The shingles vaccine is the made from the same vaccine strain and in the same way as chickenpox vaccine, except it contains a much larger amount of the vaccine virus.

For general information on vaccine additives, see Chapter 4.

How the vaccine is given

The freeze-dried vaccine is mixed with sterile distilled water and given as a single injection beneath the skin (subcutaneously). For more information on how vaccines are given, see "Getting the shot" in Chapter 4.

Schedule of vaccination

Shingles vaccine is recommended for adults over 60 years of age and may be given to people between 50 and 60 years old. At this time, only one dose is given. The need for a booster is being investigated.

Possible side effects of shingles vaccine

Local or general reactions. Pain, redness or swelling at the injection site occur in 48% of people vaccinated. Local reactions are generally mild. Rash is rare.

Reasons to delay or avoid shingles vaccine

Immunosuppression (a weakened immune system). As with all live vaccines, shingles vaccine is not usually given to people with a serious immune system disorder caused by disease or certain medications.

Shingles vaccine has been used safely in adults with mild immunosuppression. If you are immunocompromised, ask your doctor if you should receive this vaccine.

Recent injection with IG or other blood products. Although immune globulins and blood products interfere with the immune response to chickenpox vaccine, these products are not thought to interfere with shingles vaccine.

Antiviral therapy: Antiviral drugs active against varicella-zoster virus, specifically acyclovir, valacyclovir and famciclovir, make the shingles vaccine inactive. These drugs should not be taken one day before or up to 14 days after the shingles vaccine has been given.

For more information, see "Reasons to delay or avoid a vaccine" in Chapter 6.

The results of vaccination

Shingles vaccine has been shown to prevent shingles and post-herpetic neuralgia in older adults.

Snapshots

- In healthy children, chickenpox vaccine is very safe and very effective.
- Chickenpox can be a mild illness, but it can also cause severe damage and even death.
- Children who develop illness despite being vaccinated have very mild symptoms.
- Chickenpox vaccine is also effective in teenagers and adults who have not yet had chickenpox.
- Protection from one dose lasts at least 7 to 10 years. Protection from 2 doses is expected to last much longer.

- Chickenpox is a costly disease. The parents of infected children incur the largest proportion of costs.
- Shingles is a problem especially for older people, who are more likely to suffer complications and have more severe and prolonged pain than younger people.
- Shingles vaccine is safe and effective in preventing shingles in older adults.

8

Diphtheria

Diphtheria is an infection caused by bacteria called *Corynebacterium diphtheriae*. These bacteria usually infect the nose or throat. Some strains make a toxin (poison) that can severely damage the throat. The toxin can also attack the heart, nerves and kidneys.

A history of diphtheria

Before vaccine

Before 1900, diphtheria was one of the main causes of death in children. After 1900, improving socio-economic conditions helped to lower death rates for many common infections, including diphtheria. But while the death rate from diphtheria began to fall, the number of cases did not change very much. Until 1920, about 12,000 cases and 1,000 deaths occurred every year in Canada.

Treatment for diphtheria first became available in the early 1920s, which led to a further decline in death rates. Quarantining (isolation) of cases was also introduced and rigidly enforced in major cities, which helped to slow the spread of diphtheria.

After vaccine

Diphtheria toxoid, the vaccine against diphtheria, was developed in the 1920s in France and Canada. Studies of children in Ontario between 1925 and 1930 found the vaccine to be highly effective. The routine immunization of children became widespread in Canada after 1930.

In 1924, 9,000 cases of diphtheria were reported in Canada. Since 1992, there have been fewer than 5 cases reported per year, and no deaths. Diphtheria has become a very rare disease in all countries where children are immunized. Today, almost all cases of diphtheria in Canada and the United States occur in adults who have been either partially immunized or not immunized at all.

The germ

Diphtheria bacteria infect only humans.

How the germ causes illness

To cause diphtheria, the bacteria must be able to make diphtheria **toxin** (a very potent poison). The bacteria release toxin as they grow and multiply, and the toxin causes the damage. If an infected person has no protective antibodies, the toxin kills many cells lining the nose and throat.

Underlying tissues become red, swollen and painful. A thick, leathery membrane forms over the damaged area. This membrane can get so large that it blocks the airway and causes suffocation, especially if a person's larynx (voice box) and/or trachea (windpipe) are infected.

The toxin may also be absorbed into the body. It can then damage the heart, nerves and kidneys. Damage to the nerves can cause temporary paralysis.

Death from diphtheria occurs from suffocation, when the membrane blocks the airway, or from toxin damaging the heart.

Much less frequently, diphtheria causes skin infections, usually at the site of a wound or burn. Skin infections tend to be mild and without complications but they can last a long time if not recognized and treated appropriately.

How diphtheria spreads

Spread from an infected person to another person requires close contact. When an infected person coughs or sneezes, droplets containing many bacteria can land in the nose or throat of another person who is close by. When diphtheria infects the skin, the disease can spread when others touch the sores.

Healthy carriers. People who are immune to diphtheria can still carry diphtheria bacteria. That means the bacteria can infect an immune person—someone who has antibodies to diphtheria—without causing illness. These antibodies protect the person from the disease by binding to the toxin so that it cannot damage cells. However, antibodies against the toxin do not always stop diphtheria bacteria from growing in the nose or throat, making this person a "healthy carrier".

A long contagious period. The risk of spreading the disease lasts as long as diphtheria bacteria remain in the nose or throat. Most people carry

> **Healthy carriers may still be contagious**
> They can spread germs to others even though they are not ill. However, people who are ill with diphtheria are much more likely than healthy carriers to spread the infection, because they have larger quantities of bacteria in their nose and throat.

diphtheria bacteria for up to 4 weeks following infection unless they are treated with appropriate antibiotics. But some people can carry the bacteria for months. Antibiotics can promptly eradicate diphtheria bacteria by making the sick person (or healthy carrier) non-contagious.

The illness

Symptoms. The time between exposure to diphtheria bacteria and becoming sick is usually 1 to 5 days. A sore throat, loss of appetite and low fever are the first symptoms. Fever is rarely higher than 38.5°C. Within a day or two, pain in the throat becomes severe and the person is increasingly ill, weak and inactive. A person with diphtheria looks very sick.

Physical evidence. Grey-coloured patches of pus are seen in the throat. These patches may combine to form a single membrane which covers the back of the throat, tonsils and soft palate. The membrane sticks to surface tissue and cannot be easily removed. Lymph glands in the neck are very swollen and tender. The entire neck may become swollen.

Recovery. Without treatment, the membrane begins to soften and break off in pieces after about a week, and symptoms of the illness gradually disappear.

Complications

Diphtheria is a severe disease. About 1 person in 10 with diphtheria still dies even with appropriate treatment.

Suffocation. In about one-quarter of cases, the membrane in the throat extends down into the larynx and/or trachea. This form of diphtheria occurs most often in children under the age of 4. Signs of diphtheria affecting the larynx include hoarseness, noisy breathing (called "stridor") and increasingly difficult breathing. The membrane gets so big that it completely blocks the larynx, causing death by suffocation.

Heart failure. If enough toxin is absorbed into the body, it can damage the heart muscle. Heart failure and disturbance of heartbeat may occur, which can lead to death.

Nerve damage. Damage to nerves occurs in about 20% of cases. Nerves that lead to muscles are damaged more often than nerves carrying pain and other sensations. Paralysis develops 2 to 8 weeks after the illness starts. Most patients recover from paralysis caused by diphtheria toxin, but recovery can be very slow.

Kidney failure. Diphtheria toxin can also damage blood vessels in the kidneys, causing kidney failure.

Diagnosis

Tests are needed. The diagnosis of diphtheria is based on the results of throat and nose swab cultures.

Treatment

Antitoxin. If a person's symptoms suggest diphtheria, treatment starts immediately, without waiting for test results. Swabs are obtained for culture to confirm the diagnosis. Treatment requires injection of diphtheria antitoxin, which contains antibodies that neutralize or block the effects of the toxin.

How antitoxin is made

Diphtheria antitoxin is made by immunizing horses against diphtheria toxin. Some of their blood is then taken and processed. Cells are removed and the remaining liquid is partially purified to concentrate the diphtheria antibodies. Horses are used because their size permits large amounts of antitoxin serum to be prepared.

Early treatment prevents heart damage. The sooner antitoxin treatment is started, the better. If treatment begins within 48 hours of the start of illness, the death rate is about 5%. If treatment does not begin until the seventh day of illness, the death rate is 15% to 20%. Early treatment also reduces the risk of paralysis later on.

Antibiotics shorten the contagious period. Antibiotic treatment does not affect the duration or severity of the illness, because the toxin that causes the damage has already been produced and absorbed by the body by the time treatment has begun.

However, antibiotics such as penicillin or erythromycin are very effective in eliminating diphtheria bacteria from the throat. Patients with diphtheria are treated with antibiotics to shorten the time they are contagious and lower the risk of spreading the disease.

Post-recovery

People who recover from diphtheria do not always develop immunity. Diphtheria toxin is so powerful that the amount causing disease may be too small to actually stimulate the immune system. People must therefore be fully immunized after they recover from diphtheria.

The vaccine

Type of vaccine

Inactivated bacterial toxin. The vaccine against diphtheria, known as diphtheria toxoid, was developed in 1923. It was discovered that treating diphtheria toxin with small amounts of formaldehyde made the toxin harmless without affecting its ability to induce antibody. The vaccine contains inactivated (harmless) diphtheria toxin.

How diphtheria toxoid is made

Process. Diphtheria bacteria are grown in liquid culture, releasing toxin as they multiply. The bacteria are removed and formaldehyde is added to the remaining liquid to inactivate the toxin and turn it into a harmless toxoid. The toxoid is purified, concentrated and combined with alum (an aluminum salt), which enhances the immune response to the vaccine by increasing the amount of antibody produced. The final vaccine contains less than 0.02% (less than 200 parts per million) of residual formaldehyde.

For general information on vaccine additives, see Chapter 4.

Available forms of diphtheria toxoid

A combined vaccine. In Canada, diphtheria toxoid is only available in combination with one or more other vaccines. For more information, see "Vaccine types" in Chapter 4.

Vaccines for babies and young children contain 12–25 units of diphtheria toxoid per dose. Vaccines for older children and adults contain a smaller amount (only 2 units of diphtheria toxoid per dose). The reduced dose minimizes local reactions such as swelling or redness in older children and adults, who are more likely to experience local reactions with higher doses.

How the vaccine is given

Diphtheria vaccine is given by injection into muscle. For more information, see "Getting the shot" in Chapter 4.

Schedule of vaccination

Infants and children (under age 7). For routine immunization of young children in Canada, 4 doses of diphtheria vaccine (in combination with other vaccines) are given at 2, 4, 6 and 18 months. A booster dose follows at 4 to 6 years of age. If a dose is missed or delayed for any reason, the missing dose should be given but the series does not have to be started again.

Children (age 7 and over), adolescents and adults. For this group, whether as an initial vaccine or as a booster, a vaccine with a lower dose of diphtheria toxoid is used. Vaccines with a lower dose of diphtheria toxoid are also used for the booster at 4 to 6 years old in some provinces or territories.

An adolescent booster is given routinely to teens (at 14 to 16 years old).

Adult boosters. Diphtheria vaccine does not provide lifelong immunity. A booster every 10 years is recommended.

Did you know?

Many adults never get a booster shot for diphtheria. They should get *at least* one booster at age 50, and more often if they travel to an area of the world where diphtheria is not controlled.

Possible side effects of diphtheria toxoid

Diphtheria toxoid is one of the safest vaccines in use.

Local reactions. Redness, swelling, pain and tenderness at the injection site are much more common in children and adults receiving boosters of the diphtheria vaccine than in infants receiving their first 3 doses.

For more information on possible side effects after receiving the combination vaccine, see Chapter 6, Adverse events and common concerns.

Reasons to delay or avoid diphtheria vaccine

For general information on reasons to delay or avoid a vaccine or vaccines, see Chapter 6.

The results of vaccination

Diphtheria vaccine prevents disease in most children and adults who have received all of the recommended doses. People who get diphtheria in spite of being fully vaccinated have a much milder illness with fewer complications.

Diphtheria is rare, but it's still with us

Even when most children are vaccinated, the bacteria do not disappear from the population. The vaccine prevents the *disease* caused by diphtheria toxin, but does not prevent persistence of diphtheria *bacteria* in the population.

Evidence that diphtheria vaccine works:

- Diphtheria has virtually disappeared in countries where immunization of infants and children is routine.
- During outbreaks in other countries, the number of cases in fully immunized children is 85% to 90% lower than in unimmunized children.
- Immunized people who get diphtheria have milder disease and fewer complications.

> **Outbreaks prove that diphtheria could re-emerge in Canada if immunization levels decline**
>
> The efficacy of diphtheria toxoid is highlighted by the experience of Russia, Ukraine and other states of the former Soviet Union.

In Russia, Ukraine and states of the former Soviet Union, the number of children being vaccinated dropped dramatically in the late 1980s for several reasons, including large population movements and the disruption of health services, concern about adverse effects, and the use of a less effective vaccine.

This decline was quickly followed by an extremely large diphtheria epidemic: between 1990 and 1995, over 140,000 cases of diphtheria and 4,000 disease-related deaths were reported in Ukraine and Russia alone. The epidemic was eventually controlled by a mass vaccination program.

Similarly, due to inadequate vaccine coverage, 145 reported cases of diphtheria occurred in the Dominican Republic between 1997 and 2000, resulting in 36 deaths.

Snapshots

- Immunization with diphtheria toxoid has been extremely effective in preventing diphtheria.

- In Canada and the United States, most parents and doctors today have never seen a child with diphtheria. The success of routine vaccination is confirmed by the fact that fewer than 5 cases per year have been reported in Canada since 1992.
- Don't be fooled! Diphtheria bacteria have not disappeared, and the disease will return without continued routine vaccination.
- The vaccine is very safe. While local reactions sometimes occur, serious or life-threatening events caused by diphtheria toxoid are extremely rare, if they occur at all.

9

Haemophilus influenzae type b (Hib)

In spite of its name, *Haemophilus influenzae* has nothing to do with influenza (the flu). Influenza is caused by a virus, not by bacteria.

The bacteria *Haemophilus influenzae* type b (or Hib) can cause bacterial meningitis and other serious infections. Meningitis is an infection of the membranes and fluid surrounding the brain and spinal cord. Hib can also infect the epiglottis (a protective flap of cartilage in the throat), the bloodstream, lungs, joints, bones and skin. Hib infects young children. The risk of Hib disease in healthy older children and adults is very low.

In Canada, rare cases of invasive Hib still occur.

A history of Hib

Before vaccine

Before 1985, Hib caused most cases of bacterial meningitis in children, in Canada and most other parts of the world. Every year in Canada, about 1,500 cases of Hib meningitis occurred in children under 5 years old, with an equal number of other severe Hib infections. About one-half of all Hib infections occurred in children younger than 18 months old, and most were in infants aged 6 to 11 months. As much as one-third of all cases of serious pneumonia (a lung infection) in infants were caused by Hib.

After vaccine

The first vaccine against Hib was developed in the 1970s and was found to protect children over 2 years of age. Unfortunately, it did not protect most victims of this illness—children younger than 2 years old. This early vaccine was approved for use in Canada in 1986 and was recommended for use in children 2 to 5 years of age. Fortunately, subsequent research led to improved Hib vaccines that were also effective in young infants.

Before and after

- Before vaccine was available in Canada, about one child in every 300 developed Hib meningitis or another severe infection by the age of 5.
- After vaccine, no more than 16 children under 5 had Hib each year between 2007 and 2012.
- Most cases of Hib disease today involve children who have not been vaccinated.

Hib infections have almost disappeared in countries that routinely immunize infants. In Canada, the number of cases of Hib disease declined rapidly after the Hib vaccine was introduced for 2-month-olds in 1992. Between 1996 and 2004, fewer than 8 cases per year were admitted to children's hospitals—a 98.4% decrease—and numbers have remained low since then. The same decrease was seen in national surveillance data for all reported cases of Hib disease, not just in those hospitals. The largest number of cases in children younger than 5 years of age in any year between 2007 and 2012 was 16. Similar remarkable results have been seen in every country with an effective children's immunization program that includes Hib vaccine.

Not surprisingly, most cases of Hib disease today involve children who have not been vaccinated.

The germ

Hib bacteria infect only humans. Infection always starts in the nose or throat, where the bacteria attach to cells on the surface of the respiratory tract.

Healthy carriers. Healthy people can carry Hib bacteria. The bacteria can live and multiply in the nose or throat without causing any illness, especially in people who have already developed immunity to Hib. Most healthy carriers are toddlers 18 to 35 months of age, and preschool children 3 to 5 years old.

Before the routine use of Hib vaccines, most children became infected with Hib bacteria at least once in their first 5 years of life, usually through contact with other young children (e.g., a sibling or classmate in a child

What is a healthy carrier?
Children may have no symptoms after becoming infected with Hib. They become temporary "carriers" of the bacteria in their nose or throat.

care or preschool program). Some children became ill; others became carriers and eventually managed to clear the bacteria on their own.

It is not known why one child becomes a carrier while another develops serious disease. Most serious Hib illnesses occur in children younger than 5 years old. Older children and adults with certain medical conditions are also more likely to become very ill (see the text box in "Schedule of vaccination", below).

How the germ causes illness

Infection and illness. Hib bacteria have an external coat, or capsule, made of a large, complex sugar (polysaccharide). This capsule protects the bacteria against attack by white blood cells, our body's main defense against infection. If a person doesn't have antibodies to Hib, white blood cells can't attack and kill Hib bacteria. The bacteria then invade the body, multiply freely and cause disease.

While the capsule protects Hib bacteria from attack by white blood cells, another part of the wall of the bacteria, called **endotoxin**, causes the damage. When endotoxin is released into the body, it causes an intense reaction called **inflammation**. If the bacterial infection is not treated, inflammation can get out of control and cause damage throughout the body, especially to blood vessels.

Infection of the bloodstream. If the infected person has no immunity against Hib, bacteria may enter the bloodstream and infect almost any other part of the body: the brain, lungs, joints, bones, or tissues under the skin.

Meningitis is caused by bacteria infecting the membranes and fluid covering the brain and spinal cord. Inflammation can affect blood supply to the brain by obstructing blood vessels. Brain cells cannot survive interruption of their blood supply for very long, and inflammation can cause permanent brain damage.

In some children, a severe throat infection called **epiglottitis** blocks airflow to the lungs.

How Hib spreads

Hib bacteria live in mouth and nose secretions, and can be spread by healthy carriers as well as by people who are ill.

Spread from an infected person to another person requires close contact: through droplets spread by uncovered coughs and sneezes or a transfer of saliva (e.g., by kissing or drinking from a shared bottle, glass or straw).

Hib infections are **not highly contagious** and not all children who get the bacteria become sick.

Healthy carriers can spread Hib

Infected toddlers with no symptoms of illness can spread Hib by putting toys or other objects in their mouths, then sharing them with other toddlers.

The illness

The incubation period (the period between exposure and the start of symptoms) for Hib disease is not known. Illness probably occurs within a few days of being infected. Symptoms can come on suddenly (in a matter of a few hours) or gradually (over a few days).

Two kinds of infection cause symptoms.

Surface infections spread Hib bacteria along the surface of the respiratory tract (or "mucosa"), without invading the bloodstream. Surface spread can cause:
- **otitis:** an ear infection
- **sinus infections**
- **conjunctivitis:** an eye infection
- **pneumonia:** a lung infection.

Each type of infection can be caused by many other germs. Today, Hib is responsible for very few cases. That is why, for example, Hib vaccine won't prevent most ear infections, which are usually caused by pneumococcal bacteria (see Chapter 18), other strains of *Haemophilus influenzae* (not type b), and bacteria called *Moraxella*.

Symptoms of surface infections. Surface infections can produce a range of symptoms (see Table 9.1 for a summary). Fever, loss of appetite, nausea, vomiting and other general symptoms may or may not be present.

Invasive infections are uncommon but severe. Invasion of the bloodstream by bacteria (bacteremia), a very severe illness in itself, can also lead to other serious infections, such as:

- **meningitis:** infection of the membranes and fluid that cover the brain and spinal cord
- **epiglottitis:** infection of the epiglottis, in the throat
- **osteomyelitis** and **septic arthritis:** bone and joint infections.

Symptoms of invasive infections. Once Hib bacteria enter the bloodstream, fever usually develops. Other common symptoms are aches and pains, irritability, and feeling generally unwell.

- **Bacteremia** usually alters blood circulation. Endotoxin from the Hib bacteria affects blood vessels throughout the body, including the heart. Blood circulation to the skin often decreases. A child with bacteremia may be pale and cool to the touch despite having a fever. Heart rate increases. In severe cases, bacteremia can lead to shock (a life-threatening drop in blood pressure).

- The earliest signs of **meningitis** are fever and changes in consciousness or behaviour (see Table 9.2). Fever is caused by bacteremia. Brain function is disturbed by changes in the blood supply. Once the fluid and membranes covering the brain and spinal cord are infected, blood vessels going to and from the brain become inflamed. Narrow or blocked blood vessels interfere with normal blood flow to the brain.

- **Epiglottitis** is an infection of the epiglottis (the flap of cartilage covering the airway opening at the back of the throat). Infection of the epiglottis and surrounding tissue by Hib causes swelling. The swollen epiglottis blocks airflow air to the lungs. A child with epiglottitis has great difficulty breathing. This infection can develop *very* rapidly (within 4 to 8 hours). Other symptoms are fever, sore throat and drooling (because swallowing saliva is difficult).

- **Infections of a joint or bone** is another complication of Hib bacteremia. Symptoms include a sudden fever, joint or bone pain, decreased mobility, redness and swelling.

Table 9.1
Symptoms and complications of Hib, surface infections

Infected area	Type of infection	Symptoms	Complications
Ears	Otitis media	• Fever • Crying from pain	• Deafness • Chronic ear infection
Sinuses	Sinusitis	• Fever • Stuffy nose • Crying from pain	• Infection can spread from the sinus to the eye or brain and cause blindness or brain abscess • Death
Eyes	Conjunctivitis	• Fever • Redness, swelling of eyelids • Pus from eyes	• Infection can spread to the back of the eye and cause blindness or brain abscess • Death
Lungs	Pneumonia	• Fever • Cough • Rapid breathing • Difficulty breathing	• Empyema (pus surrounding the lungs) • Death

Complications

Of meningitis. Even with early diagnosis and proper treatment, Hib meningitis is a very severe disease: death occurs in about 1 out of 20 cases. Without treatment, all children with Hib meningitis die. Meningitis damages blood vessels and raises pressure within the skull, interfering with blood supply. Brain cells die quickly if their blood supply is interrupted.

About 1 in 3 survivors of Hib meningitis will have some **brain damage**, though severity varies widely. Permanent brain damage is more likely when children experience coma, seizure, paralysis or other neurological abnormalities during the acute stage of illness.

Disabilities resulting from brain damage may include developmental delay, a speech or language disorder, blindness, epilepsy and paralysis. Some level of deafness occurs in 15% to 20% of survivors; profound (total) deafness occurs in 3% to 5%.

Children who are behaving normally when they leave hospital are unlikely to develop signs of brain damage later. They may show minor abnormalities on psychological tests, but there are usually no issues with behaviour or school performance.

Table 9.2
Signs and symptoms of Hib meningitis

Earliest signs and symptoms	Later signs and symptoms

• Fever, usually high
• Significant change in behaviour such as
  - drowsiness, confusion, impaired consciousness, coma
  - irritability, fussiness, crying, agitation
  - fussiness and crying alternating with drowsiness
	• Severe headache*
	• Stiff neck or pain/tenderness on moving neck or back*
	• Not wanting to move or be moved
	• Bulging fontanelle (the soft spot on top of the skull)
	• Vomiting
	• Seizures (convulsions)

* Usually absent in babies

Of epiglottitis. This infection can happen so quickly that, without treatment, a child's airway is blocked completely, causing suffocation and death. Timely treatment with antibiotics and a tube inserted through a child's nose or mouth to bypass the swollen epiglottis and ease breathing can cure epiglottitis.

Of bacteremia. In severe cases, bacteremia can lead to shock (a life-threatening drop in blood pressure).

Of joint or bone infection. Permanent damage can happen, particularly after an infant's hip joint becomes infected. A severe bone infection can also impair normal growth.

Diagnosis

Tests are needed to diagnose Hib infections.

Surface infections. Testing a sample of pus from behind the eardrum can help to identify the specific bacteria causing an ear infection, but such tests are not routinely done. Identifying the bacterial cause of sinusitis and pneumonia also requires specific samples: fluid samples must come from the sinuses or lungs. Throat and nose cultures do not work.

Invasive infections. Diagnosis is made by detecting Hib bacteria in specimens from the patient's blood, spinal fluid, joint fluid, bone or other infected sites. Meningitis can only be confirmed by performing a lumbar puncture—inserting a small needle into the spinal canal in the lower back and removing a sample of fluid. This fluid is examined in the laboratory for bacteria and for signs of inflammation, such as more white blood cells than normal and changes in concentrations of protein and sugar.

Treatment

Antibiotics. Doctors prescribe antibiotics for bacterial ear infections, sinusitis or pneumonia. For most ear and sinus infections, antibiotics can be given by mouth. Children with pneumonia sometimes need intravenous (IV) antibiotics (given by vein) because they are too ill to take medicine by mouth.

Intravenous treatment. All invasive infections caused by Hib must be treated with high doses of antibiotics given intravenously (through an

Protecting other young children in a household

Because the incubation period for Hib disease isn't known and the timing of symptoms can vary, the risk of the bacteria infecting others in a family or household even before a serious case is diagnosed is significant.

To avoid the spread of serious illness if there are unimmunized children under 4 years old in the home, all household members are given an antibiotic called rifampin, which is taken by mouth. If all children were fully immunized with Hib vaccine before the onset of infection in the family member, rifampin is not needed.

IV drip). Early antibiotic treatment reduces the death rate of Hib meningitis by 95%. Additional treatment (e.g., for fever and seizures) may be needed, as well as IV fluids until a child is able to drink. IV antibiotics for meningitis and other invasive infections are given for at least 7 days.

Post-recovery

Children who have had a serious Hib infection don't always develop solid immunity and may be at risk of a second episode. They still need to be immunized on schedule.

The vaccine

Type of vaccine

Purified polysaccharide–protein conjugate vaccine. Hib vaccine is made from the polysaccharide capsules that protect Hib from being attacked and destroyed by white blood cells. In vaccines, they help trigger the human immune response to make antibodies. Antibodies combine with polysaccharides to coat bacteria surfaces, making it easy for white blood cells to ingest and kill them.

Because the vaccine is a highly purified extract and does not contain whole bacteria, it is impossible to get the disease or symptoms of the disease from the vaccine.

The original vaccine against Hib disease, which contained only the purified polysaccaharide, was effective in children older than 2 years of age. Children under 2 years old do not respond to vaccines containing polysaccharides alone.

Improved conjugate vaccines. A better type of vaccine was developed. This time, the purified polysaccharide was chemically linked to a purified protein, such as diphtheria toxoid or tetanus toxoid. This combined polysaccharide–protein vaccine, known as a conjugate vaccine, works for all age groups, including young infants. (Conjugate means "joined together".) The conjugate vaccines being used in Canada in 2015 have tetanus toxoid as the protein.

How Hib vaccine is made

Process. Hib bacteria are grown in liquid culture. When growth is complete, the bacteria are removed and the polysaccharide is extracted and purified. A chemical process binds the purified polysaccharide to the protein. The final product is purified and sterilized by filtration, then freeze-dried.

For general information on vaccine additives, see Chapter 4.

Available forms of Hib vaccine

Combinations. Hib conjugate vaccine can be used on its own but is usually combined with other vaccines. For more information, see "Vaccine types" in Chapter 4.

The same type of Hib vaccine is used for all age groups.

How the vaccine is given

The Hib vaccine, alone or combined with other vaccines, is given by injection into muscle. For more information, see "Getting the shot" in Chapter 4.

Schedule of vaccination

Infants and toddlers (to age 18 months). The combined vaccine is given at 2, 4 and 6 months of age, with a booster at 12 to 24 months of age.

Children between 15 months and 60 months (5 years) of age who have *not* received the Hib vaccine need only one dose.

Healthy children over 5 years of age, adolescents and adults do not receive the vaccine because the risk of Hib disease in these groups is very low.

Children age 5, adolescents and adults at higher risk of invasive Hib disease need one dose, regardless of whether or not they received the Hib vaccine before age 5 years.

> **Medical conditions that increase risk of invasive Hib disease**
>
> - Sickle cell disease and certain other congenital disorders of hemoglobin (red blood cells)
> - Absent spleen or a spleen that does not work well because of a congenital defect, disease or surgery
> - Conditions or treatments that weaken the immune system, including congenital conditions, cancer, HIV infection, transplantation of bone marrow, stem cells or an organ transplant
> - Cochlear implants (including children who are to receive implants)

For more information on people at increased risk, see Chapter 3, When extra protection is needed.

Boosters (to enhance prior vaccinations). After the primary booster at 12 to 24 (usually 18) months of age, further booster doses are not necessary.

Long-lasting protection. After primary immunization in infancy and the booster at 12 to 24 months of age, protection lasts for many years. Primary immunization builds immune memory: a person's immune system can make specific antibody promptly when exposed to Hib bacteria later in life.

Possible side effects of Hib vaccine

Hib vaccines are extremely safe. When given as a separate injection, Hib conjugate vaccines cause local redness and pain in 5% to 15% of infants.

The addition of the Hib vaccine to combination vaccines does not increase the frequency or severity of side effects. Put another way, side effects from the combination vaccines are the same with or without the addition of Hib vaccine.

For more information on possible side effects after receiving a combination vaccine, see Chapter 6, Adverse events and common concerns.

Reasons to avoid or delay Hib vaccine

For general information on reasons to delay or avoid a vaccine or vaccines, see Chapter 6.

The results of vaccination

Rates of Hib meningitis, epiglottitis and other severe Hib infections have dropped dramatically in Canada and other countries where infants routinely receive Hib vaccine. Within only 2 years of starting routine infant vaccination against Hib in Canada, Hib disease had become a rare occurrence.

A child vaccinated against Hib is protected in two ways:
• Immunity prevents Hib bacteria from invading the bloodstream.
• Immunity prevents Hib infection from becoming established in the nose and throat. With fewer healthy children carrying Hib bacteria, the spread of Hib has decreased dramatically.

Having less Hib spreading around also indirectly protects:
• Infants younger than 2 months old, who are too young to be vaccinated.
• Immunocompromised children and adults, who may not respond well to the vaccine.

This indirect effect, called "herd immunity" occurs only when almost all children are vaccinated.

> **Two kinds of protection**
>
> Hib vaccine protects the child who is immunized *and* decreases spread of Hib among children generally—an important indirect effect.

Evidence that Hib vaccine works:
• Controlled trials have shown that the vaccine prevents meningitis and other serious Hib infections.

- The frequency of Hib meningitis and other serious Hib infections has declined dramatically in all countries where Hib vaccine was added to the routine infant schedule.
- After introducing Hib vaccine in Canada, the rate of Hib meningitis and other serious Hib infections declined by 99% in 12 children's hospitals with active programs to detect and monitor all such infections.
- Studies confirm that not only is Hib *disease* disappearing, but Hib *bacteria* are also disappearing as a result of routine vaccination. It is not yet known whether routine vaccination will eventually lead to total eradication of Hib bacteria.

Snapshots

- Hib infections cause severe illness, especially in children under 5 years old.
- Even with treatment, invasive Hib infections can cause death or severe disabilities.
- The Hib vaccine, given alone or in combination with other vaccines, is very safe and effective.
- Hib disease is disappearing from every country where infants are routinely vaccinated against Hib.

10

Hepatitis A

Hepatitis A is one of several viruses that can infect the liver. The liver is the body's main chemical factory:
- It completes food digestion, which starts in the stomach and intestines. The liver changes the food into forms that can be used by various body tissues.
- It stores sugar, fat and certain vitamins.
- It breaks down many chemicals and toxins so that they can be excreted by the body.

Many people infected with hepatitis A do not know they have the virus because they do not get sick. This is especially true when young children are infected. But infected people with no symptoms are still contagious and can spread the virus to others.

People who do get sick after infection with hepatitis A may have fever, fatigue, loss of appetite, nausea, vomiting, and yellow skin and eyes (called "jaundice"). Usually, it takes weeks to recover. Only rarely is the infection so severe that it causes death.

Unlike hepatitis B virus, hepatitis A does not cause chronic infection.

A history of hepatitis A

Before vaccine

The number of hepatitis A infections in Canada and the United States has declined over the past 40 years, as socio-economic conditions, especially community hygiene and sanitation, have generally improved. Hepatitis A infection is more common in children than in adults.

The risk of infection with hepatitis A virus is higher in the following groups:
- Travellers to or immigrants from poor or under-resourced parts of the world, where sanitation is substandard and transmission rates are high (e.g., Latin America, Central America, Africa, Asia, Oceania and parts of Eastern Europe).
- People living in rural or remote areas with no access to clean water or adequate sanitation (e.g., some First Nations reserves).
- Residents and workers in correctional institutions or facilities caring for the developmentally challenged.
- People with lifestyle risks for infection, including users of oral or injectable illicit drugs, and men who have sex with men.
- Household or close contacts of someone with acute hepatitis A.
- Household or close contacts of a child adopted from a country where hepatitis A is common.
- People with hemophilia who use plasma-derived blood products.

After vaccine

Hepatitis A vaccine was approved for use in 1995 in Canada but has not yet been recommended for routine use.

Controlled studies have shown that the vaccine is very safe and very effective in preventing hepatitis A infections. Since the hepatitis A vaccine was introduced in Canada in 1996, the number of cases reported annually has declined by over 90%.

In the United States, hepatitis A vaccine was recommended in 1996 for people at higher risk of infection and for all children in communities with high rates of infection. In 1999, children in states (and counties) with high rates of hepatitis A infection were added. By 2003, there had been a 88% drop in infections in states and counties that routinely vaccinated. In 2006, hepatitis A vaccine was recommended for *all* children 12 to 23 months of age.

The actual number of hepatitis A cases is thought to be seven times higher than the number reported, because infected people are often not tested for the virus.

The germ

Hepatitis A virus is a member of the large family of viruses called picornaviruses. Other members of this family include polioviruses, enteroviruses, and the common cold virus (rhinovirus).

How the germ causes illness

Liver infection. After the virus is swallowed, it passes through the stomach into the intestinal tract. Hepatitis A is an especially hardy virus and is not affected by stomach acids. It multiplies first in cells of the intestine and then spreads to the blood, where it remains for up to 2 weeks before the onset of illness. The virus then infects the liver.

Virus produced within the liver is excreted into bile and reaches the intestinal tract. From there, it is shed in the stool.

How hepatitis A spreads

Infants and young children with a hepatitis A infection usually have no symptoms at all. But they are just as contagious as people who become ill.

Fecal contamination. The virus usually spreads from person to person and can be found in the stool of an infected person for as long as 21 days before symptoms appear until 8 days after they start. People infected with hepatitis A are most contagious from about 2 weeks before to 7 days after symptoms begin, when the concentration of virus in the stool is highest.

Hepatitis A usually spreads by contact with an infected person who hasn't done thorough handwashing after going to the bathroom. The virus can be transmitted by contact with an infected person, or by food, utensils or surfaces that have been touched with contaminated hands. The virus can easily spread during a diaper change, when virus picked up on the hands is inadvertently carried to the mouth.

A hardy virus that spreads easily

The ability of the hepatitis A virus to survive for weeks in the environment adds to the ease of transmission. It can live for weeks in water (both fresh and salt), moist soil and live shellfish.

Young children are important spreaders of hepatitis A infection. They often have no symptoms, are not yet able to perform appropriate hygiene, are likely to contaminate their surroundings, and require lots of hands-on care.

Hepatitis A also spreads through **contaminated food** and, less often, by **contaminated water**. Community outbreaks in Canada have been linked to infected food handlers.

Only rarely has the virus spread through contaminated blood products.

The illness

When infants and young children do get sick, which only happens about 30% of the time, their illness is usually mild and brief, with fever but no jaundice. Often a child's infection isn't recognized as hepatitis until an older family member develops jaundice.

Older children, adolescents and adults are much more likely to become ill when infected. Their symptoms may include fever, fatigue, loss of appetite, nausea, vomiting, abdominal pain and jaundice. The illness can last several weeks, but most people recover completely. About one-quarter of infected adults require hospitalization.

Complications

Occasionally, the liver damage from hepatitis A is so severe that the infection is fatal (in 1 to 3 per 1,000 cases). Severe liver failure may require an emergency liver transplant. Unlike hepatitis B, hepatitis A virus does not cause chronic infection of the liver, cirrhosis (scarring of the liver) or liver cancer.

Diagnosis

Because many different viruses can cause the same symptoms as hepatitis A, **a blood test is needed** to identify the infection. The test finds specific antibodies produced in response to hepatitis A virus, which are present by the time jaundice occurs.

Treatment

There is no specific treatment for hepatitis A. Bedrest is recommended only as long as a person feels too ill to be out of bed.

Post-recovery

Immunity after infection is life-long.

The vaccine

Type of vaccine

Killed intact virus vaccine. The vaccine cannot cause hepatitis A infection or symptoms because it does not contain live virus.

How hepatitis A vaccine is made

Process. The virus is grown in tissue culture cells, extracted, purified and then killed with formaldehyde. Three different vaccines are available in Canada. The manufacturing process differs slightly among formulations, as does the dosing.

For general information on vaccine additives, see Chapter 4.

Available forms of hepatitis A vaccine

Alone or in combination. Hepatitis A vaccine is available as a single vaccine or in combination with hepatitis B or typhoid fever vaccine.

In general, the combined hepatitis A and hepatitis B vaccine should be given to children, adolescents and adults who need protection against both viruses. (Hepatitis B is another virus that infects the liver. For more information, see Chapter 11.)

The combined hepatitis A and typhoid fever vaccine is available for people aged 16 years and older, and may be used for travellers who need protection against both infections. For more information on travel vaccines, see Chapter 3, When extra protection is needed, and the Appendix to this book.

Young children. Three hepatitis A vaccines and the combination vaccine (hepatitis A and hepatitis B) are approved for use in Canada in children one year of age and older. Hepatitis A vaccine may be given to children as young as 6 months of age if risk of exposure is high.

Older children and adults. The same vaccines are used, but higher doses are given to adolescents and adults. The age at which a higher dose is recommended varies with the type of hepatitis A vaccine.

How the vaccine is given

Hepatitis A vaccine is injected into muscle. For more information, see "Getting the shot" in Chapter 4.

Schedule of vaccination

Travellers. One dose of hepatitis A vaccine is enough to provide 6 to 12 months of protection for a traveller going into an area where hepatitis A infection is common.

> **The children of newcomers to Canada may need this vaccine**
>
> Children born in Canada to parents who grew up in a country where hepatitis A is common are usually not immune to the virus, although their parents likely are. These children should get hepatitis A vaccine before visiting their parents' country of origin.

The combined hepatitis A-typhoid fever vaccine is given in a two-dose schedule, with the second dose 36 months after the first.

General. For long-lasting protection, 2 doses, given 6 to 36 months apart, are recommended for children aged 1 year and older, adolescents and adults.

Infants less than one year of age. If a first dose is given at less than one year of age, 2 further doses are needed for long-lasting protection.

The combined hepatitis A-hepatitis B vaccine can be given in a two-dose schedule (second dose 6 to 12 months after the first) or a three-dose schedule (second dose at one month and third at 6 months after the first dose).

Boosters. It is not yet known whether booster doses of hepatitis A vaccine will be needed, but it is expected that protective antibody levels will last for at least 20 years.

Who should get hepatitis A vaccine?

- Travellers to countries with high rates of hepatitis A, including non-immune immigrants returning to visit their home countries*
- Immigrants from countries with high rates of infection, unless they are already immune
- Household or close contacts of a child adopted from a country where hepatitis A is common
- Children and adults living in areas of Canada where hepatitis A infection is common (e.g., some Aboriginal communities)
- People who have chronic liver disease from any cause (including hepatitis C or B)
- People with hemophilia treated with products made from plasma
- People with lifestyle risks for infection, including illicit drug use and men who have sex with men
- Military personnel and relief workers likely to be posted to areas with high rates of hepatitis A
- Workers involved in research on hepatitis A virus or production of the vaccine
- Zookeepers, veterinarians and researchers who handle non-human primates
- Anyone who wishes to be protected against hepatitis A vaccine

---

*For more information, see "Vaccines for travellers" in Chapter 3, and the Appendix to this book

Preventing hepatitis A after exposure: Post-exposure control

Vaccine

Hepatitis A vaccine is given to:

- Non-immune people sharing a household or having other close contact with a person with hepatitis A
- Contacts in a group child care centre or kindergarten program
- Co-workers and clients of a food handler with hepatitis A infection.

Hepatitis A vaccine is not routinely given to school or other workplace contacts unless there is an outbreak. It should be given as soon as possible and preferably within 14 days of last exposure. Effectiveness after that time is unknown. Treatment with immune globulin (IG) may also be required.

Passive immunization: Immune globulin

In addition to hepatitis A vaccine, immune globulin (IG) may be needed to protect exposed people. IG contains large amounts of antibodies against hepatitis A, providing immediate protection against infection.

- **Immune globulin alone** is given to infants younger than 1 year of age who have been exposed to hepatitis A within the previous 14 days. The vaccine may be less effective in this age group.
- **Immune globulin** should also be used when vaccine is contra-indicated or unavailable.
- **Immune globulin** *and* **vaccine** are required for individuals who are immunocompromised (their immune system does not function well).
- **Vaccine alone** is sufficient for most people (older than 1 year) who have been in close contact with hepatitis A within the previous 14 days, unless they have a condition that affects immune function.

IG is given by injection into muscle.

> **If an exposure to hepatitis A occurred more than 2 weeks ago...**
>
> Neither vaccine nor immune globulin is known to be effective. Vaccine may still be given, especially in a household or other close setting where the virus may be circulating and further exposures may occur.

How is IG made? Immune globulin is obtained from the plasma (the liquid part of blood) of volunteer donors who have large amounts of antibody against hepatitis A.

Is IG safe? Current methods of testing blood from volunteer donors and of preparing IG ensure that there is no risk of acquiring HIV, hepatitis B, hepatitis C or any other known virus from this product. Other than pain at the injection site, there are almost no significant reactions to IG. Rarely, allergic reactions have been reported.

Possible side effects of hepatitis A vaccine

Other than mild pain and redness at the injection site, side effects are uncommon. Because the vaccine is a killed virus, it is not possible to get the infection from the vaccine.

The results of vaccination

Hepatitis A vaccine has been 85% to 90% effective in preventing illness with hepatitis A. Immunity is expected to last for many years after vaccination.

Evidence that hepatitis A vaccine works:
- In a large controlled trial of children in Thailand who received 2 doses, hepatitis A vaccine was 94% effective.
- In a smaller controlled study in New York, protection was 100% after only one dose.
- Vaccinating children in U.S. states with high infection rates reduced the number of infections by 88% between 1999 and 2003.

- Using the vaccine during community outbreaks has brought spread of the disease under control. The vaccine also prevents spread within households.

Snapshots

- Hepatitis A virus is excreted in feces and spreads by close contact with an infected person or by ingesting contaminated food or water. Young children are important spreaders of this infection.
- While infection is common in young children, they do not often get sick. Older children and adults are much more likely to become ill when infected.
- Hepatitis A does not cause chronic liver disease, but infection may cause liver failure and even death.
- Hepatitis A vaccine contains no live virus, and is very safe and effective.
- At present in Canada, hepatitis A vaccine is given to selected high-risk children and adults, to control outbreaks, and to prevent infection after exposure. Even this limited use of the vaccine had reduced the number of cases of hepatitis A in Canada by 90% between 1996 and 2012.

11

Hepatitis B

Hepatitis B is an infection of the liver caused by the hepatitis B virus. The liver is the body's main chemical factory:

- It completes food digestion, which starts in the stomach and intestines. The liver changes the food into forms that can be used by various body tissues.
- It stores sugar, fat and certain vitamins.
- It breaks down many chemicals and toxins so that they can be excreted by the body.

One-half of people who are infected with hepatitis B do not know they have the virus because they do not get sick. They have an "asymptomatic" infection (no symptoms). Of this group, 10% of adults and 90% of newborns are unable to get rid of the virus naturally (i.e., their immune system cannot do the job by itself). Because these people don't know they have the disease, they don't seek treatment and remain infected for life.

They become "chronic carriers" of hepatitis B, and may develop liver disease or liver cancer after many years of infection with this virus.

The other half of infected people become ill with fever, fatigue, loss of appetite, and yellow skin and eyes (called "jaundice"). The illness may last weeks or months. Severe liver damage caused by infection may be fatal. Most people recover from the acute infection and are immune for life, but some become chronic carriers.

> **Hepatitis B is global**
>
> Hepatitis B is one of the most common and serious infectious diseases in the world. About 5% of the world's population are chronic carriers of HBV, and nearly 25% of all carriers develop serious liver disease, causing more than one million deaths every year.

A history of hepatitis B

Before vaccine

The illness called hepatitis was described by Hippocrates more than 2,000 years ago. Studies done during World War II showed that there were at least two different types of viral hepatitis. They were originally called infectious hepatitis and serum hepatitis, but are now called hepatitis A and B. (See Chapter 10 for information on hepatitis A.)

Chronic carriers. About 300 million people worldwide are chronic carriers of hepatitis B virus (i.e., the virus is in their body, but no symptoms appear for many years). The frequency of this type of infection varies widely around the world.

Before vaccination began, about one person in 200 (0.5%) was a chronic carrier of hepatitis B infection in Canada, the United States and some other developed countries. In present-day China, Southeast Asia and parts of Africa, an estimated one person in 10 (10%) is a chronic carrier. In these countries, the most common way of way of getting hepatitis B infection is at birth, when the virus is passed from an infected mother to her newborn. The risk of becoming a chronic carrier is highest in newborns infected by their mothers.

In Canada, it has been estimated that 20,000 new hepatitis B infections (including both symptomatic and asymptomatic) occurred every year before 1982, when the first vaccine became available. Up to 10% of these infections resulted in chronic infection of the liver. Every year, chronic hepatitis B infection caused about 400 deaths from cirrhosis (scarring) of the liver and about 80 deaths from liver cancer.

In Asia and other parts of the world where the rates of hepatitis B infection are higher, cancer of the liver caused by hepatitis B is the most common type of cancer.

After vaccine

The first hepatitis B vaccine became available in 1982. Subsequent changes to how the vaccine was made led to widespread availability and considerable reductions in cost. These newer vaccines were licensed in Canada in 1987.

Hepatitis B vaccine has been shown to be very safe and very effective in preventing infection with hepatitis B virus.

In Canada, use of the hepatitis B vaccine has expanded over time:
- 1982: people at high risk of exposure or of severe disease begin to receive the vaccine.
- 1987: screening for all women in pregnancy and the vaccination at birth of infants of infected mothers are recommended.
- 1991: routine immunization of all children before adolescence is recommended.
- Early 1990s: school-based programs begin.

School programs have been a great success, both in reach—well over 90% of eligible children—and effect. From 1990 to 2008, the reported rate of new hepatitis B infections in children 10 to 19 years of age declined by 90%.

Hepatitis B immunization is now routine throughout Canada, though not on a universal schedule. In some provinces and territories, the vaccine is given to infants starting at 2 months of age; in others, it is given in primary school. Both schedules are effective.

The average number of new infections reported each year has decreased from over 3,000 in 1990 to 582 in 2008. The number of infants being infected by their mothers at birth is also decreasing because *all* expectant mothers are now tested for the illness. A baby born to an infected mother can be protected immediately after birth with hepatitis B immune globulin (HBIG) and vaccine.

In other countries, mass immunization of all newborn infants in countries with high rates of chronic hepatitis B infection, such as China, Korea, Taiwan and Thailand, has been extremely effective. By 2006, 162 World Health Organization countries had introduced hepatitis vaccine into their routine infant immunization programs. Not only has the rate of infection of young children decreased by over 90%, but the rates of liver cancer caused by hepatitis B infection and deaths from overwhelming hepatitis in infants have also declined markedly.

Did you know?
Hepatitis B vaccine was the first vaccine shown to prevent cancer in humans.

The germ

The hepatitis B virus has an outer protein coat, called hepatitis B surface antigen (HBsAg for short), and an inner core protein that covers the DNA genes of the virus. Immunity to hepatitis B virus depends primarily on a person's antibody response to HBsAg.

How the germ causes illness

After infecting the liver cells, what happens to the hepatitis B virus depends on the body's immune response to it. In a healthy response, immune white blood cells attack the infected liver cells and destroy them. In the process, the virus is also destroyed.

Chronic liver infection. Some people infected with hepatitis B do not have the normal immune response to the virus and are unable to get rid of the infected cells. The virus survives and continues to multiply in liver cells, causing a chronic infection.

Eventually, this chronic infection damages the liver, which may lead to scarring (known as **cirrhosis**) and death from liver failure.

Chronic infection can also cause **cancer of the liver**, which is almost always fatal. Newborns infected at birth have the highest risk of developing liver cancer later in life. Many years may pass between the infection and onset of illness due to chronic liver disease. During this time, a person may not be aware of the infection because no symptoms develop.

How hepatitis B spreads

Body fluids. Chronic carriers remain contagious for as long as the virus is in the liver, usually for life. For chronic carriers and people acutely ill with hepatitis B, the virus is present in their blood and certain other body fluids, including semen and vaginal secretions. Other body fluids that become contaminated with blood may also have hepatitis B virus in them (see Table 11.1).

Table 11.1
The most common ways that hepatitis B virus spreads

Means of infection	Examples
The linings of the mouth or genital tract are exposed to blood or body fluids containing blood, or to genital secretions	• A newborn exposed to an infected mother's blood before or during birth • Sexual activity or intimate physical contact with an infected person • Sharing personal hygiene items that may be contaminated with blood (e.g., a toothbrush) with an infected person
Penetration of the skin with virus-contaminated equipment	• Injection with a contaminated needle or syringe • Tattooing and body piercing with contaminated equipment • Hemodialysis (filtering of the blood) with contaminated equipment or fluids • Sharing razors or other sharp items
Transfusion	Blood, platelets or plasma containing hepatitis B virus

In Canada, the two most common means of spread today are sexual activity and needles shared by illicit drug users. The infection rate is highest among older teenagers and young adults.

Since the 1970s, all blood products used in Canada are screened to make sure that they are free from hepatitis B. Also, all needles and syringes used by health care personnel are for single use only. However, blood may still be the source of infection for people with hepatitis B who have come to Canada from countries where blood screening resources or injection equipment are less available.

The illness

The incubation period (the time between infection and start of symptoms) for hepatitis B varies between 6 weeks and 6 months. This is much longer than the incubation period of most other infections.

Symptoms of acute illness. About one-half of people infected with hepatitis B develop an acute illness and experience symptoms for up to a week before jaundice appears. Symptoms include fever, headache, aches and pains, loss of appetite, nausea and vomiting, and skin rash (red spots scattered over the body). Most people feel weak and tired.

Jaundice is sometimes the first sign of illness. A person's urine looks darker. Over the next few days, the skin and whites of the eyes turn yellow, and bowel movements usually become light brown or grey.

Recovery. The illness is usually mild in children. The duration of illness can vary widely, from a few days to many weeks. Jaundice and other symptoms gradually clear. Most older children, adolescents and adults infected with hepatitis B virus make a complete recovery, develop lifelong immunity and do not get chronic liver disease.

Chronic carriers. Some people, whether they have symptoms or not, are unable to get rid of the virus and become chronic carriers. They risk spreading the disease to others and may develop **chronic liver disease** later in life.

Complications

Acute infection. In about 1 out of 100 acute infections, the illness is so severe that the liver stops working altogether. The risk of death is high.

Chronic infection. The most common complication is persistent infection of the liver or chronic hepatitis, which can be asymptomatic for years.

Eventually, loss of appetite, weight loss, abdominal pain, fluid retention and bleeding problems may develop because of liver damage. Chronic infection over time often leads to **cirrhosis** (scarring of the liver), which can cause liver failure and death. Chronic infection with hepatitis B virus can also cause **liver cancer**. About 25% of people with untreated chronic infection eventually die of liver failure or liver cancer.

Diagnosis

Blood tests can confirm abnormal liver function and infection with hepatitis B virus. Blood tests are also needed to detect a chronic hepatitis B infection.

Blood screening. Sensitive and accurate blood tests developed in the 1970s enabled the routine screening of blood donors for hepatitis B virus. A rapid and marked decrease in hepatitis B infections associated with the transfusion of blood and blood products followed.

Treatment

There is no treatment for acute hepatitis B infection. Various medications are now available to treat **chronic hepatitis B** infection and help protect against liver damage, but they are not always successful.

Post-recovery

Immunity after recovering from hepatitis B and clearance of carriage is believed to be life-long.

The vaccine

Type of vaccine

Purified viral protein vaccine. Hepatitis B vaccine is made from the protein that forms the outer coat of the virus particle. The protein is highly purified and contains no other part of the virus. The vaccine cannot cause hepatitis B infection or symptoms because there are no whole virus particles in the vaccine.

Hepatitis B vaccine is unique. Unlike the other vaccines discussed in this book, hepatitis B vaccine was developed even though the virus itself cannot yet be grown in the laboratory.

How hepatitis B vaccine is made

Process. The vaccines currently used in Canada are prepared by recombinant (meaning "formed by recombination") gene technology. The gene that makes the hepatitis B surface protein is isolated and transferred into yeast cells. The yeast cells act like factories: as they multiply, they make large quantities of hepatitis B surface protein. The protein is extracted from the fluid culture that the yeast is grown in, then purified. The vaccine contains less than 50 mg (0.05 g) of yeast protein per dose. The yeast cells cannot make whole virus or any other part of the virus except the surface antigen.

For general information on vaccine additives, see Chapter 4.

Available forms of hepatitis B vaccine

Alone or in combination. Hepatitis B vaccine is available as a single vaccine or in combination with other vaccines.

A combined vaccine containing hepatitis B, diphtheria, tetanus, pertussis, polio and Hib vaccines is available for routine immunization of infants and young children. This is the vaccine usually given to infants.

A combined vaccine containing hepatitis B and hepatitis A vaccines is useful for travellers going to parts of the world where these infections are common. For more information on travel vaccines, see Chapter 3, When extra protection is needed, and the Appendix to this book.

When hepatitis B vaccine is given as a single vaccine, the same products are used for infants, older children and adults, but the dosage (amount injected) varies with age, product and (for children 11 to 15 years old) whether 2 or 3 doses are used. A larger dose is given in two-dose schedules.

How the vaccine is given

Hepatitis B vaccine is injected into an arm or leg muscle. For more information, see "Getting the shot" in Chapter 4.

Schedule of vaccination

There is no universal schedule for giving hepatitis B vaccine in Canada. The vaccine is routinely given to infants, pre-teen schoolchildren, or both.

The most common schedule (for all ages) is 3 doses of vaccine given over a 6-month period. The second dose is given 1 month after the first dose; the third 5 months later.

Infant hepatitis B immunization programs are in place in many provinces and territories, especially since the combined vaccine became available in 2004.

School immunization programs for pre-teen children are in most provinces and territories. A two-dose schedule, which has been shown to be just as effective as the standard three-dose schedule in this age group, is used in school programs.

Programs for immunizing high-risk individuals are in place in all provinces and territories (see text box, opposite). Non-immune people at high risk should be vaccinated as soon as the risk is recognized, regardless of age. This means that children may be vaccinated at an earlier age than is routine. People with a weakened immune system or renal failure need higher doses of hepatitis B vaccine.

Pregnant women are routinely screened for hepatitis B and all newborns of infected mothers are immunized shortly after birth, ideally within 12 hours, and again at 1 and 6 months of age. Premature infants weighing less than 2,000 grams at birth receive an extra dose of vaccine at 2 months of age.

Boosters (to enhance prior vaccinations). Protection after hepatitis B vaccination lasts for many years, if not for life. Immune memory ensures lasting protection even after antibodies against hepatitis B disappear from the blood.

Booster doses are usually not recommended except for some people with an underlying health condition that interferes with normal immune responses. (See Chapter 3, When extra protection is needed.)

Whether or not boosters will be needed by children vaccinated in infancy is not yet known and is being evaluated.

People at high risk for hepatitis B

- All newborns of mothers with hepatitis B infection
- Individuals with a health condition that makes them more likely to be exposed to hepatitis B (e.g., disorders requiring infusions of blood, blood products or hemodialysis)
- Individuals with a health condition that could make a hepatitis B infection more severe (e.g., a weakened immune system or chronic liver disease)
- Household and other close contacts of an acute hepatitis B case OR a known carrier
- Adolescents and adults with lifestyle-related exposures to blood or body fluids (e.g., unprotected sexual activity or the injection of illicit drugs)
- Children and workers in any child care setting where a child (or co-worker) has acute hepatitis B OR is a known carrier
- Families in communities where hepatitis B is considered endemic (e.g., some First Nations and Inuit communities)
- Immigrant or refugee families from countries with high rates of hepatitis
- Travellers to countries with high rates of hepatitis, including immigrants returning to visit their home countries
- Families adopting a child who has tested positive for hepatitis B
- Adolescent and adult residents of, or workers in, occupations with potential exposure to blood or body fluids (e.g., health care, facilities for the developmentally challenged, correctional institutions and testing laboratories)

Preventing hepatitis B after exposure: Post-exposure control

Vaccine

Hepatitis B vaccine is given to unimmunized or partially immunized people to prevent hepatitis B. It should be given as soon as possible and preferably within 7 days of exposure. Hepatitis B immune globulin is given as well.

Hepatitis B vaccines are **safe during pregnancy** and should be given without delay if a non-immune woman is exposed to infection. Acute hepatitis B infection can cause severe disease during pregnancy and chronic infection in an unborn child.

Passive immunization: Immune globulin

If a non-immune person is exposed to hepatitis B virus, a special preparation of immune globulin, called **hepatitis B immune globulin (HBIG)**, is used to prevent infection. HBIG is injected into muscle and contains a high concentration of antibody against hepatitis B virus. The antibodies coat the virus particles, enabling white blood cells to destroy the virus before it can damage the liver.

Does HBIG work? For best results, HBIG is given as soon as possible after exposure, preferably within 48 hours. Its effectiveness is unknown if given after 7 days. HBIG is about 75% effective in preventing infection.

How is HBIG made? HBIG is prepared from the plasma (the liquid part of blood) of volunteer donors who have high concentrations of antibody against hepatitis B.

Is HBIG safe? Current methods of testing blood from donors and of preparing HBIG ensure that there is no risk of acquiring HIV, hepatitis B or hepatitis C or any other known virus from this product. Other than pain at the injection site, there are no significant reactions to HBIG.

Who should be treated with HBIG?

- Newborns whose mothers are infected with hepatitis B
- Non-immune children or adults who receive an accidental needle-stick injury with a needle previously used for injection or a splash of blood into the mouth or eye
- Non-immune people who have engaged in sexual activity with an infected person
- Non-immune people who have shared injection equipment with an infected person

---

Possible side effects of hepatitis B vaccine

Mild, local and temporary. About 15% of people getting this vaccine experience mild pain and tenderness at the injection site, lasting less than 24 hours. Carefully controlled studies have found that general symptoms, such as fever, headache, muscle aches and pain, nausea, vomiting, loss of appetite and fatigue, occur at the same rates in people who receive the vaccine as in those who are given a placebo (in this case, an injection containing no vaccine).

Allergic reactions are rare, occurring after less than 1% of vaccinations, and may be caused by an allergy to yeast proteins in the vaccine.

For more information on possible side effects after receiving the combination vaccine, see Chapter 6, Adverse events and common concerns.

Safe vaccine. Millions of doses of hepatitis B vaccine have been given over the past 30 years. The various hepatitis B vaccines have been shown to be very safe. There is no risk of infection with hepatitis B or any other virus from the vaccine.

Unfounded claims. There have been rumours in the past that hepatitis B caused multiple sclerosis (MS). There is no valid scientific evidence of a relationship between this vaccine and MS. Nor are patients with MS at risk of exacerbating their symptoms by receiving hepatitis B vaccine.

Reasons to delay or avoid hepatitis B vaccine

For general information on reasons to delay or avoid a vaccine or vaccines, see Chapter 6.

The results of vaccination

In general. Hepatitis B vaccine is very effective. Over 95% of people who are vaccinated develop antibody and are protected against infection with hepatitis B virus. Individuals who become infected despite vaccination are protected against developing chronic hepatitis B infection. Protection lasts many years, if not for life.

First Canadian strategy. When the vaccine first became available in 1982, it was recommended for groups considered to be at higher risk of infection with hepatitis B. While this early strategy was very effective in reducing the rate of infections in target groups, there was little or no effect on the overall rate of hepatitis B infections in the decade that followed. That's because many people in the high-risk groups were still not vaccinated, and many chronic carriers did not know they were infected.

Current strategy. To control hepatitis B infection in the general population, programs to immunize all pre-adolescents, before they became sexually active, began in the early 1990s. Since then, programs to immunize all infants were started in several provinces and territories. The United States and many other countries routinely vaccinate all infants.

The rationale for Canada's current strategy

The decision to recommend hepatitis B vaccination for all children was based on three main facts:

- The vaccines, whether given alone or in combination, are safe and effective.
- School-based vaccination programs are efficient and affordable.
- It costs much more to treat chronic liver disease caused by hepatitis B than to vaccinate all children.

Evidence that hepatitis B vaccine works:
- Controlled trials have shown that giving hepatitis B vaccine to newborns whose mothers are infected is over 95% effective in preventing infection of the newborn.
- Controlled trials have also shown that hepatitis B vaccine is over 90% effective in preventing infection by means of sexual transmission.
- The long-term benefits of routinely vaccinating all infants have been proven in Taiwan. There, rates of infection in newborns and older children have dropped significantly, along with rates in liver cancer caused by hepatitis B infection.
- The routine immunization of schoolchildren has lowered rates of new hepatitis B infections in adolescents in several Canadian provinces and territories.

Snapshots

- Hepatitis B disease is a major health problem world-wide: more than 3 million people have chronic infection.
- Chronic liver disease and liver cancer resulting from hepatitis B infection cause many deaths world-wide.
- Hepatitis B vaccine is very safe and effective.
- Hepatitis B vaccine was the first vaccine shown to prevent cancer in humans.
- The routine vaccination of children offers the opportunity to eradicate hepatitis B and prevent a common type of cancer.
- School vaccination programs in Canada have been very successful, reaching over 90% of eligible children.
- Now that a combination vaccine is available, infant vaccination programs are becoming routine.

12

Human papillomavirus

Papillomaviruses are a large group of viruses that infect many different mammals, including humans, cattle, dogs, rabbits, horses, deer and elk, among others. Diseases caused by human papillomaviruses (HPVs) are a major health problem throughout the world. HPV infections are very common. In fact, almost everyone will be infected with HPV during their lifetime.

The most serious diseases caused by HPV are cervical cancer, and cancers of the penis and the anus.

There are over 100 different strains of HPVs, in two main groups: one group infects the skin; the other infects cells that make up the surface of the mouth, genital tract and anal tract.

Because HPVs cannot be grown easily in the laboratory, relatively little was known about them until the 1970s. Since then, advances in molecular biology have made it much easier to identify HPV genes in tissue and recognize diseases caused by HPVs.

A history of HPV

Before vaccine

HPV infection is the most common sexually transmitted disease. And while most infections cause no detectable illness, HPV-related diseases can also take two main forms: cancers and warts.

Cancers. HPV infections are a leading cause of cancers of the genital tract, anal tract and mouth. Cervical cancer, which kills an estimated 250,000 women every year worldwide, is the most common form. About 80% of cervical cancer cases occur in women in less developed countries, where it is the number-one cause of cancer in women.

The first study suggesting that HPV infection caused cervical cancer was reported in 1975. By the early 1980s, several strains of HPV had been isolated: some were linked to genital warts and others to cervical cancer. Recent studies have found that HPV is present in 99.7% of cervical cancers.

Every year in Canada, about 1,300 women are diagnosed with cervical cancer and 350 die of the disease. An estimated 220 women also die each year of vulvar and vaginal cancers caused by HPV infection. Fortunately, screening programs with Pap smears have been very successful

> ### HPV infection is very common
> Almost everyone is infected with HPV at some point in their lifetime, including about 3 of every 4 sexually active Canadians. The peak risk for HPV infection is within 5 to 10 years of the first sexual experience. People 20 to 24 years of age have the highest rates of infection, but teenagers also have high rates of infection.

in reducing the death rate from cervical cancer in Canada and other developed nations.

In men, HPV infection is a factor in about 90% of anal cancers and 50% of penile cancers.

HPVs also cause genital **warts**, common skin warts, and warts affecting the airways of infants.

After vaccine

HPV infections can be prevented by a vaccine, which causes the body to produce antibodies against proteins that make up the external coat of the virus. These antibodies are specific to the types of HPV contained in the vaccine, and cannot protect against other types.

One HPV vaccine was approved for use in Canada in 2006 and a second vaccine in 2010. Studies show that both vaccines are very effective at preventing infection and pre-cancerous changes in the cervix. They can also prevent HPV infections in boys and men.

The germ

Of the more than one hundred types of HPVs, only 16 cause cancer. Two of these 16 cause over 70% of all cervical cancers.

The disorders caused by different types of HPV are listed in Table 12.1.

Table 12.1
Diseases associated with human papillomavirus infections

Disease	HPV types	Method of spread
Cervical cancer	16, 18, 45, 31 and others	Sexual contact
Anal and penile cancer	16, 18	Sexual contact
Anogenital warts	6, 11	Sexual contact
Recurrent papillomatosis of the respiratory tract in newborns and infants	6, 11	Mother to child, at birth
Skin warts	1, 2, 3, 4, 10 and others	Non-sexual contact

How the germ causes illness

HPVs infect surface cells either of the skin or mucous membranes. HPVs do not spread beyond the surface but cancer cells produced by HPV infection can spread through the body.

Skin and genital tract. Some strains infect the skin and cause common warts. Others infect the surface cells of the genital tract and cause cervical cancer, genital warts, anal cancer or cancer of the penis.

Rarely, a newborn baby can become infected during birth if a mother has active HPV infection of the birth canal. The infant develops an infection of the respiratory tract, which can spread from mouth to trachea.

Cancer and warts. Usually, HPV infections are brief, have no symptoms and are quick to disappear. Occasionally, however, the virus lives on in infected cells, causing them to develop into cancerous cells or a wart.

How HPV virus spreads

Sexual transmission and skin-to-skin contact. HPV infections spread from person to person during sex causing genital warts and infections of the cervix or other sites in the genital tract or in the mouth. Sexual transmission happens during vaginal intercourse, anal intercourse and oral sex. The HPV types that cause genital warts can be transmitted by skin-to-skin contact and do not require intercourse for spread. Common skin warts spread from person to person by direct skin-to-skin contact with warts.

Very contagious. HPV infections are extremely common and occur soon after a person first engages in sexual activity with an infected partner. HPV infections of the genital tract are especially contagious.

> **HPV infections are very contagious**
> Sexual contact with one infected person is estimated to cause the virus to spread to two-thirds of later sexual partners.

The illness

Most infections of the genital tract remain latent, meaning there are no signs of infection and no illness develops. Genital warts are the most common result of HPV infection of the genital tract.

Cervical cancer. Most infections with cancer-associated types of HPV are also latent. But if infection persists because a person's immune system is unable to get rid of the virus, there is a high risk of developing cancer.

Infections with persistent high-risk HPV types lead first to **cervical intra-epithelial dysplasia (CIN),** a change in the infected cervical cells that is detectable by Pap smear. CIN is an early stage in the development of cervical cancer. Typically, the sequence leading from infection to cervical cancer happens in five stages over many years:

1. The cervical epithelial (surface) cells are infected by a cancer-causing HPV type, usually in a person's late teens to early twenties.
2. The immune system can't eliminate the virus, leading to persistent infection.
3. Minor abnormalities become detectable on Pap smear (at 20 to 30 years of age).
4. More serious changes (e.g., CIN) or cancer localized to surface tissues occur (at 30 to 40 years of age).
5. Invasive cancer of the cervix (at 40 to 60 years of age).

HPV can also cause cancer of the vulva and vagina in women, cancer of the penis in men, and cancer of the anus in both sexes.

Anogenital warts in the anus/vagina/penis area are also called genital warts or condylomas. They are the most common disorder caused by genital HPV infections. About 1% of sexually active men and women 18 to 49 years of age have external genital warts. But warts can appear on the upper thighs and in folds of the groin as well as inside the vagina, on the cervix, within the urethra, or in and around the anus. Most genital warts are caused by HPV-6 and HPV-11, which almost never cause cervical cancer.

Skin warts are common in school-age children and adolescents. They decrease as we age, probably because the developing immune system gets better at resolving this kind of infection. Skin warts do not lead to cancer.

Diagnosis

Genital warts and skin warts are diagnosed by examination. Laboratory tests are not required, except for Pap smear testing of the cervix to identify HPV-associated cervical disease.

Pap smears are an excellent screening test for the early pre-cancerous lesions of HPV infection. Regular screening with Pap smears should begin within 3 years of first intercourse and no later than age 21.

Treatment

HPV is treated by destroying or surgically removing HPV-infected tissue. Treating cervical cancer requires some form of surgery, with radiation therapy or chemotherapy, or both in cases of advanced disease. Warts can be surgically removed, destroyed with caustic chemicals or frozen with liquid nitrogen.

Post-recovery

How long protection lasts after recovering from an HPV infection is not known.

The vaccine

Type of vaccine

HPV vaccines are called **virus-like particle (VLP) vaccines**.

How the HPV vaccines are made

HPV vaccines are **recombinant vaccines.** (Recombinant means "putting genes together".) The gene for the protein that makes up most of the external coat of the HPV particle (called the L1 protein) is inserted into yeast cells or into insect tissue culture cells.

These culture cells act like tiny factories, making large amounts of L1 protein, which is then extracted and purified. The purified protein forms into round particles, called "virus-like particles" or VLPs. They carry the L1 protein but are empty spheres. They do not contain any live virus, and therefore cannot cause infection.

Although HPV grows poorly in the laboratory, VLPs can be made in very large amounts in yeast or cell cultures.

For general information on vaccine additives, see Chapter 4.

Available forms of HPV vaccine

Inactivated vaccine. Two different vaccines have been developed:
- Cervarix (HPV2) contains VLPs made from HPV-16 and HPV-18, the two most common causes of cervical cancer. It is a bivalent (meaning "two-in-one") vaccine.
- Gardasil (HPV4) contains HPV-16 and HPV-18 as well, but also includes HPV types 6 and 11, the most common causes of genital warts. This is a quadrivalent ("four-in-one") vaccine.

Both HPV vaccines are recommended for girls and women. Only HPV4 is recommended for immunizing boys and men.

A new "nine-in-one" vaccine that protects against an additional five types of HPV that more rarely cause cancer was licensed in Canada in early 2014. It is too soon to know how it will be used.

How the vaccine is given

Both vaccines are given by injection into muscle. For more information, see "Getting the shot" in Chapter 4.

Schedule of vaccination

Adolescent girls and young women. Both HPV vaccines are recommended for girls and women 9 to 26 years of age. For best results, *all* girls need to be vaccinated at 9 to 13 years of age, well before they become sexually active.

The vaccine may also be given to unvaccinated women 27 years of age or older who are at ongoing risk of exposure to HPV for life-style or other reasons.

After receiving the HPV vaccine, girls and women who are sexually active still need regular medical exams, including Pap smears, because of rare cases caused by other HPV strains.

Education is needed

Ideally, *all* children should be vaccinated between 9 and 13 years of age, well *before* the age at which sexual activity begins, as part of a school-based vaccination program.

However, many parents (and teens) in Canada don't know very much about HPV. They may not realize that the infection spreads during sex or that it causes cancer. Parents may be reluctant to see their child as a sexually active being and not recognize the need for this vaccine.

The ultimate success of HPV vaccine will depend on universal school-based programs and public education.

Adolescent boys and young men. HPV4 is recommended for boys and men 9 to 26 years of age. For best results, *all* boys should be vaccinated at 9 to 13 years of age, well before they become sexually active.

The vaccine may be given to unvaccinated men 27 years of age or older who are at ongoing risk of exposure to HPV for life-style or other reasons.

Which type of HPV vaccine to choose depends upon whether protection against genital warts is needed. If so, vaccination with HPV4 is recommended. If the goal is to prevent cancer, either vaccine can be used.

Three doses of either vaccine have usually been given: the first dose between the ages of 9 and 13, the second dose 1 to 2 months later, followed by the third dose 6 months after the first dose.

A two-dose schedule for girls and boys 9 to 14 years of age has been recently introduced in Canada.

Booster doses. How long the vaccine protects against HPV is not yet known, so whether boosters will be needed is also unclear.

Possible side effects of HPV vaccine

Mild to moderate pain and swelling at the injection site are common.

Adolescents and young adults sometimes faint after being given the HPV vaccine. This reaction can also happen when they are given other vaccines and is thought to be caused by anxiety and pain rather than by the vaccine itself.

Reasons to delay or avoid HPV vaccine

For general information on reasons to delay or avoid a vaccine or vaccines, see Chapter 6.

The results of vaccination

Studies show that HPV vaccines are highly effective in preventing infection by the virus types contained in the vaccines. They stimulate a strong immune response. More than 99% of people who get immunized develop antibody to the HPV types in the vaccine after completing the three-dose series.

Evidence that HPV vaccine works:
- In women 16 to 26 years old, HPV4 vaccine protection against HPV types 16- and 18-related cervical disease is nearly 100%. Protection against external genital lesions caused by HPV types 6, 11, 16 or 18, including genital warts, is 95% to 99%.
- In women 24 to 45 years of age, HPV4 vaccine protected against persistent infection and cervical or external genital disease in 91% of recipients.

- In men 16 to 26 years old, HPV4 vaccine protection against HPV types 6, 11, 16 or 18-related external genital lesions is 84% to 100%; efficacy against persistent vaccine-type related infections is 70% to 96%.
- In women 15 to 25 years old, HPV2 vaccine protection against HPV types 16 and 18 is 95% to 99%.
- Studies suggest that vaccinating against HPV may prevent transmission.

Snapshots

- In healthy adolescents and young adults, HPV vaccines are very safe and very effective.
- While most HPV infections cause no symptoms, HPV remains a leading cause of genital warts and cervical cancer.
- HPV vaccines prevent persistent infection and pre-cancerous changes in the cervix from HPV types 16 and 18, which cause more than 70% of cervical cancer cases. They are also very effective in preventing genital warts caused by HPV types 6 and 11.

13

Influenza

The influenza virus causes epidemics of flu, bronchitis (an infection of the airways) and pneumonia (an infection of the lungs) *every year* in the late fall and winter. These illnesses often look like colds, but the influenza virus is much more dangerous. It can cause severe illness and even death.

Up to 20% of people are infected with influenza virus every year. No other virus causing acute respiratory illness can spread so rapidly to a large population.

Whenever outbreaks of influenza occur, more infants (babies under 12 months old) and adults age 65 and over are hospitalized. Death rates also rise during influenza outbreaks, mostly in the elderly and people who have serious heart or lung disease.

Influenza also causes **pandemics**. Pandemics happen when the influenza virus changes dramatically and is able to infect everyone worldwide because no one is immune. The new virus spreads rapidly around the world, infecting people of all ages, and may cause more severe disease and more deaths than would normally occur in seasonal epidemics. There have been 5 pandemics in the past 125 years, the latest in 2009. Existing vaccines will not work for the new virus, so a new vaccine must be produced.

The influenza vaccine is usually called "the flu shot".

A history of influenza

Before vaccine

Influenza virus was first isolated in humans in 1933. Because of its unique ability to infect many people over a short period of time, influenza has been identified in historical records as having caused 299 epidemics between the years 1173 and 1875.

A worldwide pandemic was first described in 1580. As international travel increased, so too did the spread of influenza. Major pandemics have occurred in:
- 1889–90 ("Russian Flu", with an estimated 250,000 deaths in Europe, and a death total worldwide of two or three times that number);
- 1918 ("Spanish Flu", with 20 million deaths worldwide);
- 1957 ("Asian Flu", with 2 million deaths worldwide);

- 1968 ("Hong Kong Flu", with one million deaths worldwide);
- 2009 ("swine flu", with about 280,000 deaths worldwide).

Influenza vaccine first became available in the late 1940s.

After vaccine

Every year, influenza infects 10% to 20% of North Americans. Between 4,000 and 8,000 people die from their illness each year in Canada—over 90% of whom are 65 or older.

Early influenza vaccination programs in Canada and the United States targeted high-risk groups, meaning people more likely to get very sick because of age or an underlying medical condition (see Table 13.1, "Priorities for influenza vaccination", below). These programs reduced hospitalization rates by 50% to 70% and deaths in the elderly by about 85%.

Starting in 2014–15, vaccinating all individuals over 6 months of age was recommended in Canada.

The goal of most public influenza vaccination programs in Canada still is to reduce influenza deaths and severe illnesses in high-risk people: the elderly, the very young and people of any age with a chronic medical condition. Throughout Canada, influenza vaccine is available at no cost for:
- Young children and people over 65 years of age,
- People with certain chronic medical condition, and
- People who may spread influenza to others at high risk of severe illness.

Children under 5 years old are at higher risk of complications from influenza (such as high fever, convulsions and pneumonia). Most provinces and territories now provide flu vaccine free of charge to all children in this age group; others provide it for babies 6 to 23 months old only.

At time of writing, only Ontario provides free vaccine to all residents. Whether or not vaccine will be provided free of charge for all age groups in other provinces and territories has yet to be determined.

> **The flu vaccine is free for many**
> - Influenza vaccine is now recommended for everyone 6 months of age and older.
> - Throughout Canada, influenza vaccine is available at no cost for anyone who is at high risk of serious illness and for their close contacts.

Because influenza virus changes continually and immunity to any one strain does not last long, the influenza vaccine must be given *every* year *before* the start of the flu season, which in Canada extends from the late fall to early spring.

The germ

Influenza A strains are more common. There are two main types of influenza virus: group A and group B. Influenza A strains cause most infections and all large flu epidemics. They are divided into subtypes on the basis of two proteins on the surface of the virus, called hemagglutinin (H) and neuraminidase (N).

Immunity against influenza. Immunity to these two surface proteins, especially to H, protects against infection and reduces the severity of illness when infection does occur. A person infected with one subtype of influenza A develops immunity to just that one subtype, with little or no protection against other subtypes and none at all against influenza B strains.

Almost every year, the proteins that coat the **influenza A** virus change slightly as a result of mutations in the genes for H and/or N. Even minor changes pose a problem for the human immune system, which doesn't always recognize the virus or may not respond very effectively. That is why infection with influenza can occur in the same person again and again, year after year.

Similar changes occur in **influenza B strains**, but more slowly. In recent years there have been two strains of influenza B in circulation each year.

Changes leading to global pandemics. The influenza A virus has another way of protecting itself from attack by the human immune system, called "**antigenic shift**". Here, influenza A viruses acquire an entirely new and different H or N gene, usually from an avian (bird) strain of influenza A.

Wild birds are a natural source of influenza viruses and fortunately, many bird strains do not cause infections in humans. The bird strains must mutate many times before they can infect humans and spread from person to person.

When a new H or N protein differs completely from the surface proteins on strains that have infected the population in the past, no-one is immune to the new strain. Such changes can lead to pandemics of influenza.

An ever-changing virus

The ability of the influenza virus to keep changing the proteins on its surface is key to its success in causing epidemics. Immunity to influenza is strain-specific and strains change slightly every year. Essentially, because no one person can establish very effective immune memory to the virus, it spreads through populations like wildfire.

H5N1 and H7N9—avian influenza. Over the past several years, outbreaks of an often fatal form of influenza have been reported both in wild birds and in domestic ducks and chickens. These outbreaks are caused by a strain of bird influenza called H5N1. They started in Hong Kong, but by mid-2006 had spread to most countries in Asia and into Africa, the Middle East and Europe. Migrating wild birds and the trade of infected poultry helped to spread avian influenza ("bird flu").

While H5N1 is highly contagious in birds, it has not infected humans very often. By 2014, just over 650 human infections in 16 countries had been reported to the World Health Organization. This virus causes an extremely severe pneumonia in humans: about 60% of cases have been fatal. Almost all human cases were in people exposed to infected domestic poultry. Spread from one infected person to other people has been very rare.

In 2013, a new form of fatal avian influenza (H7N9) was reported in China and, later, in other countries in Southeast Asia. As with H5N1, spread from person to person is rare.

Neither of these viruses has yet been transmitted in North America.

Vaccines against H5N1 and H7N9 are being developed in case these strains mutate into forms that do spread readily from person to person.

How the germ causes illness

The respiratory tract is the major target of influenza virus. After infected droplets are inhaled or reach the nose or eyes on contaminated fingers, the virus infects and multiplies in the surface cells lining the nose and back of the throat. The virus kills these cells. The lining of the nose, throat, trachea (the airway connecting the larynx or voice box to the bronchi), bronchi (large air passages of the lungs) and bronchioles (small divisions of the larger bronchi) are damaged to varying degrees.

How influenza spreads

The kind of illness caused by influenza virus ensures that it spreads widely. Large amounts of infectious virus are produced by infected cells and released into secretions in the nose, throat and lungs. An infected person sends virus-containing droplets into the air by coughing, sneezing, talking or singing, where they are breathed in by other people nearby. ("Nearby" means within about one metre of an infected person.)

Influenza also spreads when respiratory secretions containing virus contaminate hands, surfaces (such as a doorknob) or objects (such as a toy). The virus is picked up by others who touch hands, objects or surfaces, then touch their own eyes or nose.

Highly contagious, easily spread. Influenza spreads easily. In some cases, the illness is relatively mild and is often not recognized as influenza in school-age children or healthy young adults, who continue to go to school or to work even though they are very contagious. An infected person is contagious for 3 to 5 days after the illness starts.

The illness

Incubation—the time between exposure and the start of symptoms—is short for influenza: only 1 or 2 days. Influenza can cause a wide range of illnesses:

- A common cold-like illness with or without fever
- Typical "flu" with sudden fever, headache, aches and pains, fatigue, sore throat and cough
- High fever (greater than 40°C) without other symptoms, especially in young infants
- Croup (fever, a barking cough, difficulty breathing) in children under 2 years old
- Fever, vomiting, abdominal pain and diarrhea, with or without respiratory symptoms, especially in infants and young children.

Sudden onset. Influenza is unique for the suddenness with which symptoms start. A person can feel perfectly well, and within a few hours be overcome by headache, aches and pains, and intense fatigue.

Influenza damages the respiratory tract, causing runny nose, sore throat and cough. But more general symptoms, such as headache, aches and pains, fatigue and physical exhaustion are not the result of spread of the virus through the body. Rather, they are an intense response by the body's immune system as it tries to fight infection.

Complications

Pneumonia (an infection of the lungs) is the most common complication of influenza, caused either by the virus itself or by bacteria invading areas damaged by the virus. Pneumonia causes the most deaths from influenza, especially in people with a chronic heart or lung condition.

Other complications include the following:
- **Febrile seizures** (caused by high fever) in infants and young children
- **Myositis** (severe muscle inflammation) in children, especially with influenza B infection, usually affecting the calf muscles in both legs
- **Myocarditis** (inflammation of the heart muscle), which may lead to abnormal heart rhythm, heart failure and death
- **Encephalitis** (inflammation of the brain), which may lead to brain damage and death
- **Reye's syndrome,** a condition that damages the brain and liver. Reye's syndrome was more common when children with influenza were treated regularly with aspirin, which is thought to precipitate it for reasons that are not known. This disorder became quite rare after it was recommended *not* to give aspirin to children to control fever. Acetaminopen (Tylenol, Tempra) does not have this effect.

Diagnosis

Laboratory testing may be needed to confirm a diagnosis because influenza symptoms are so similar to other respiratory viruses. Different tests are used:
1. Rapid methods that find viral proteins or genes in respiratory secretions within a few hours are now used by most hospitals and testing centres.
2. The virus can be grown in culture from samples obtained by nose or throat swabs or by suctioning respiratory secretions. This method takes 3 to 7 days.

A quick diagnosis of influenza infection can be important for timely response:
- If a person is severely ill or at high risk of developing severe disease, medications targeting influenza can be started early.
- Control measures to reduce virus spread can be implemented, especially in hospitals, nursing and retirement homes, and other institutions that care for the elderly.

Treatment

Two types of antiviral drugs are available to treat influenza infections, if needed. Both restrain the virus from multiplying in the body. The older drug, amantadine, stops influenza A viruses from entering into healthy cells. It has no effect on influenza B strains. The newer anti-influenza drugs, oseltamivir and zanamivir, block the neuraminidase (N) protein of the virus and prevents the virus from spreading from one cell to others. They are active against both A and B strains of influenza.

Amantadine and oseltamivir are given by mouth. Zanamivir is given through an inhaler.

Timely treatment with antivirals can reduce:
• the time a person has fever and respiratory symptoms by about 50%;
• the amount of virus in respiratory secretions; and
• the period of contagiousness, helping to control spread of the virus

> **Not everyone who has influenza needs medication...**
> ...but antivirals should be used for people with severe disease or who are more likely to have a serious or complicated infection.
>
> **To have the best effect, treatment must be started within 48 hours of starting symptoms.**

Using antivirals to prevent influenza *is* recommended for some people at risk of serious illness or death from the virus. They may have already received the seasonal flu vaccine but have an underlying medical condition that makes the vaccine less likely to be effective. However, using antivirals for a long time or giving them to many people to prevent infection is *not* recommended, because the virus develops resistance.

Post-recovery

Influenza infections occur over and over in the same person. Symptoms may be milder after recurrent infections with similar viruses, but immunity does not last very long and virus strains change frequently.

The vaccine

Types of vaccine

Two types of influenza vaccines are available in Canada:
- **Inactivated (killed) virus vaccines,** and
- **A live virus vaccine** with attenuated (weakened) strains of influenza virus.

The live vaccine has two big benefits:
- It is given as a nasal spray rather than by injection.
- It works better in young children than the inactivated vaccine.

Because the H and N proteins of influenza virus are always changing, the strains used to make vaccines must be updated annually. The World Health Organization has a network of laboratories around the world to help isolate and identify current changes in influenza viruses.

The decision about which strains to include in the yearly vaccine is made in February. This may seem early, but vaccine manufacturers need enough time to produce the vaccines for the following fall and winter.

The inactivated and live influenza vaccines contain the same virus strains. Before 2014, influenza vaccines contained two strains of influenza A and one of influenza B. In 2014, vaccines containing two strains of influenza A and two strains of influenza B became available in Canada.

Why a yearly flu shot?

People need to be revaccinated every year to maintain immunity against influenza because:

- The protective effects of this vaccine only last a short time. Immunity from the vaccine, like immunity from the disease, lasts only 6 to 12 months.
- Influenza viruses are continually changing.

Why immunity lasts such a short time after influenza and most other viruses that cause colds and respiratory infections is not known.

How inactivated influenza vaccine is made

Process. Influenza viruses are grown in fertilized chicken eggs. Tens of millions of eggs are used each year to produce vaccine in Canada and the United States alone. There are several different preparations of inactivated influenza vaccine, including vaccines with three or four virus strains. While production methods vary somewhat among manufacturers, the virus is always inactivated chemically, concentrated, then purified by physical processes such as centrifugation or chromatography.

The inactivated but still intact virus particles are broken into smaller pieces to produce a **split virus vaccine**, then purified to remove almost all of the internal virus components and egg materials. These vaccines contain tiny amounts of egg protein.

Each strain of influenza is grown and processed separately, then they are combined.

Remember!
The inactivated vaccine does not contain live virus and cannot cause the flu.

Additives. Some influenza vaccines come from the manufacturer in vials containing multiple doses. These vials sometimes contain very small amounts of thimerosal (less than 0.05 mg/dose). Thimerosal is a mercury-containing preservative that helps prevent bacterial contamination of the vaccine. While there is *no evidence* that this very small amount of mercury causes any harm, thimerosal-free vaccines are also available. Some forms of influenza vaccine contain an adjuvant, which is a substance that increases the immune response to the vaccine.

For general information on vaccine additives, see Chapter 4.

How live attenuated influenza vaccine is made

Process. For each subtype in the vaccine, a weakened strain was made by growing the virus in chicken eggs at low temperatures. The virus is thus adapted to grow only in the nose, where the temperature is lower, but not elsewhere in the body. Each year, the adapted strains are then combined with the selected circulating influenza viruses. The resulting laboratory viruses contain the two surface proteins (H and N) of the wild strains, which stimulate immunity, but are otherwise made of proteins from the weakened strain. The new virus strains are then grown in fertilized chicken eggs, concentrated, purified and combined.

This vaccine contains no thimerosal. For general information on vaccine additives, see Chapter 4.

Available forms of influenza vaccine

Both the inactivated and live attenuated influenza vaccines are available in Canada.

- **Infants and young children (6 months to 2 years old)** are given inactivated vaccine. Live vaccine is not recommended for this age group because of an increased risk of wheezing.

  A vaccine with an adjuvant (a substance that increases immune response) has recently become available in Canada. It is too early to know how it will be used.

- **Children and adolescents (age 2 to 17).** The live attenuated vaccine *or* the inactivated vaccine may be used. The live attenuated vaccine is preferable for children under 6 years old because it works better than the present inactivated vaccine. Whether it also works better in older children is not yet known.

- **Adults.** Inactivated vaccine *or* live attenuated vaccine can be given to adults before age 60. Only the inactivated vaccine is licensed for older adults. The inactivated vaccine works better than the live attenuated vaccine in adults and is preferred for people with a chronic health condition. A vaccine with an adjuvant may be used for people 65 years of age and older. A high dose inactivated vaccine is also expected to be available for this age group soon.

Much research is underway to find influenza vaccines that work better and for longer, against a virus which is continually changing. New forms of flu vaccine may become available in the near future.

How influenza vaccines are given

The inactivated flu vaccine is usually injected into muscle.

The live attenuated vaccine is given as a nasal spray, using a special device. For more information, see "Getting the shot" in Chapter 4.

Who should receive influenza vaccine?

Target groups. While vaccine is recommended for everybody, public health programs in Canada to date have concentrated on vaccinating the following groups:
- People at risk of serious illness or death from influenza due to age or an underlying health condition,
- People who could spread influenza to people at risk (e.g., health care workers, the household contacts of vulnerable people, and out-of-home caregivers for children under 5 years old),
- Workers providing essential community services during influenza epidemics (e.g., ambulance drivers, police and firefighters), and
- Other designated at-risk workers (e.g., those culling poultry infected with bird influenza.

See Table 13.1, below, for details.

In the general population. Children under 5 years old and the elderly are more likely to be hospitalized with influenza. However, seasonal influenza in otherwise healthy children and adults is not only widespread but also very costly, both for families and the health care system. Most infections are still spread by children in child care, schools or other educational institutions.

Another goal of immunization is to reduce the spread of influenza. Starting in the 2014–15 season, **the National Advisory Committee on Immunization recommends yearly influenza vaccination for everyone 6 months of age and older.** Priority should still be given to people listed below.

Table 13.1
Priorities for influenza vaccination

People at high risk of severe influenza or hospitalization

- A child, adolescent or adult with any of the following health conditions:
  - a heart or lung disorder (including bronchopulmonary dysplasia, cystic fibrosis and asthma)
  - diabetes (type 1 or 2) or other metabolic disease
  - cancer or other diseases or treatments which weaken the immune system
  - chronic kidney disease
  - chronic anemia or hemoglobinopathy
  - a condition that makes it hard to control respiratory secretions or increases risk of aspiration (e.g., difficulty swallowing)
  - severe obesity
  - a child or adolescent with a condition treated for a long period of time with aspirin (e.g., arthritis)
  - a child or adolescent with a chronic neurologic disorder

- All children 6 to 59 months of age
- People of any age who live in nursing homes or other chronic care facilities
- All people ≥65 years of age
- Healthy pregnant women
- First Nations and Inuit peoples

People who could spread influenza to others at high risk (listed above)

- Health care and other care providers in facilities and community settings for people at high risk of severe influenza
- All household contacts of people at high risk of severe influenza
- All household contacts of infants under 6 months old (who are at high risk of hospitalization for influenza but too young to be vaccinated)
- All members of a household expecting a newborn during the influenza season
- Providers of child care for children under 59 months of age, whether in or out of the home
- Service providers in a close community setting where there may be people at high risk (e.g., a cruise ship)

Other workers

- People providing essential community services
- People involved with culling poultry infected with bird influenza

Schedule of vaccination

Infants younger than 6 months old don't get the flu vaccine. Current vaccines do not stimulate an adequate antibody response in young infants.

Babies and children 6 months to 9 years of age who have never had a dose of flu vaccine receive 2 doses, given *at least* 4 weeks apart, unless they have received one or more doses of vaccine in a previous influenza season; in that case, they need only one dose.

Children 9 years of age and older, adolescents and adults need only one dose of vaccine, regardless of their influenza vaccination history.

The dose of vaccine is the same for all age groups.

Short-term protection only. Immunity against the influenza virus lasts less than a year and may last less than 6 months. Optimally, the influenza vaccine should be given every year in the fall, just before the flu season begins.

Possible side effects of influenza vaccines

Common effects

Inactivated vaccine. About two-thirds of people who get the inactivated vaccine have some pain at the injection site (a local reaction) for 1 to 2 days. Up to 12% of children have a mild fever but fever is rare in adults. Other general reactions, such as muscle aches and pains, and fatigue lasting 1 to 2 days, occur even less often.

Live attenuated vaccine. Most people have no reaction to the live attenuated vaccine. Mild nasal congestion and a runny nose may happen.

Rare effects

Guillain-Barré syndrome, a neurologic disorder with muscle paralysis, has been reported after influenza vaccination. In recent years, the risk for this syndrome has been estimated to be only one additional case above the background rate (meaning the rate in unvaccinated people) for every one million influenza vaccinations. The risk is really very small.

The risk of Guillain-Barré syndrome after an influenza infection is *much* higher.

Oculo-respiratory syndrome (ORS). During 2000–01, there were 960 reports in Canada of a new adverse event occurring after influenza vaccine. The symptoms of ORS developed 2 to 24 hours after vaccination and included red eyes, respiratory symptoms (e.g., cough, sore throat, difficulty breathing, wheezing or chest tightness), and facial swelling.

These symptoms were mild and cleared within 48 hours in most cases. Less than 10% of ORS cases were in children. Three-quarters of cases were in women 30 to 59 years old. The cause of ORS is not known but is thought to be an inflammatory reaction to some component of the vaccine. With changes to the manufacturing processes, there have been only a few cases of ORS since 2001.

Reasons to delay or avoid influenza vaccine

Inactivated influenza vaccine is safe

Egg allergy is no longer considered a reason not to get this vaccine. Influenza vaccine is grown in chicken eggs and may contain minute traces of egg protein. Multiple studies have shown that inactivated vaccine is safe for people with an egg allergy.

Pregnant or breastfeeding women. The inactivated influenza vaccine is safe for women at all stages of pregnancy and for breastfeeding mothers. They should get the flu shot to protect themselves and their infant.

Oculo-respiratory syndrome (ORS). People who experienced ORS symptoms (see above) after a previous dose of influenza vaccine can still be vaccinated. If breathing problems were severe, ask your doctor if you should get the vaccine. This reaction is very rare with current vaccines.

People who have experienced Guillain-Barré syndrome (GBS) within 6 weeks of a previous dose of influenza vaccine should not get the vaccine again, unless another cause for this illness was found.

Live attenuated vaccine

People with an egg allergy. The live attenuated vaccine is not given to people who have had anaphylaxis after eating eggs. The vaccine's safety has not yet been studied in this group.

Pregnant or breastfeeding women. The live attenuated vaccine is not given to pregnant women. It has not been studied in this group and the inactivated vaccine is safe and effective. The live attenuated vaccine can be given to women who are breastfeeding.

People with immunosuppression (weakened immune function). As with all other live virus vaccines, the live attenuated influenza vaccine is not given to people who have a serious immune system disorder caused by disease or certain therapies.

People who receive live attenuated influenza vaccine should avoid close contact for 2 weeks with someone who has a very severe immune compromising condition (e.g., a recent bone marrow transplant recipient who is in hospital and requires protective isolation). There is a theoretical risk of transmitting the vaccine virus and causing infection in the transplant recipient.

Children receiving long-term aspirin therapy. Influenza infection has been associated with an increased risk of Reye's syndrome in children on aspirin therapy. Reye's syndrome has not been reported in connection with the live influenza vaccine but because of a possible risk, the live vaccine should be avoided.

People who have experienced Guillain-Barré syndrome (GBS) within 6 weeks of a previous dose of influenza vaccine should not get the vaccine again, unless another cause for this illness was found.

Live attenuated vaccine should be delayed or replaced by the inacti-vated influenza vaccine for:
- People with severe asthma who have received oral or high-dose inhaled steroids or have experienced wheezing in the past 7 days.
- People who have received antiviral drugs effective against influenza (amantadine, oseltamivir, zanamavir) in the past 2 days. Also, these drugs should not be given for 2 weeks after receiving the vaccine, because they will make the vaccine ineffective.

For general information on reasons to delay or avoid a vaccine or vac-cines, see Chapter 6.

The results of vaccination

When the strains of virus in the yearly influenza vaccines match preva-lent circulating strains, the flu vaccine prevents infection in about 70% of healthy children and adults. When people become infected despite vaccination, their illness is milder than in people who haven't had their flu shot.

Although flu vaccines are less effective in people over 65 years old than in younger adults, they still reduce severity of illness in this age group. In vaccinated elderly people, hospitalization for influenza is 50% to 70% lower and influenza-related deaths are about 85% lower, compared with those who are unvaccinated in this age group.

The routine vaccination of women in pregnancy protects them against influenza infections, protects their newborns from influenza, and lowers the risk of premature delivery and low birth weight.

Evidence that influenza vaccine works:
- Reduced influenza infection and illness rates in vaccinated children and adults.
- Reduced hospitalization rates in vaccinated children under 5 years of age.
- Reduced hospitalization and death rates in vaccinated people age 65 years and older.

- Lower influenza rates in vaccinated health care workers during influenza epidemics.
- Lower influenza rates in residents of long-term care centres when health care workers are immunized.

Snapshots

- Influenza is a highly contagious virus that can cause severe illness and even death.
- Influenza vaccine is very safe and effective. Unfortunately, it is least effective in people age 65 and over—one of the groups most at risk from influenza. However, illness is usually much milder in seniors who become infected despite being vaccinated.
- New influenza vaccines must be developed each year to match the ever-changing composition of the virus. Vaccines that provide immunity one year may not work the next year.
- The routine vaccination of groups at higher risk of severe disease or death from influenza is the most effective way to reduce the impact of yearly influenza epidemics.
- All Canadian provinces and territories have programs to provide influenza vaccine to elderly people, young children, and people with high-risk conditions regardless of age.
- In 2014 the National Advisory Committee on Immunization recommended influenza vaccination for everyone over 6 months of age.
- Searches are underway for a better vaccine, one that does not have to be given every year and which could be given to everyone. If such a vaccine can be produced, yearly epidemics of influenza may become a thing of the past!
- New forms of influenza vaccine may become available in the near future.

14

Measles

Measles is a severe illness caused by a virus. It causes high fever, runny nose, cough, conjunctivitis (pink eye or inflammation of the eyelid), and a rash lasting 1 to 2 weeks. Complications of measles occur in about 10% of cases, and often include ear infections, croup (infection of the throat and larynx [or "voice box"]), pneumonia (infection of the lungs), or diarrhea.

Encephalitis (intense inflammation of the brain) occurs in about one of every 1,000 cases, and often results in permanent brain damage. Measles causes death in about 1 to 2 of every 1,000 cases. In very rare cases, a severe and always fatal brain disease called SSPE (subacute sclerosing panencephalitis) develops years after a person has had measles.

A history of measles

Before vaccine

Measles was recognized as a distinct infection in the early 17th century. Most of its features were described by a Danish physician, Peter Panum, during an epidemic on the Faeroe Islands in 1846. He confirmed that measles is contagious and found that the interval between exposure and the start of the rash is 14 days. He also observed that infection results in lifelong immunity: elderly people living on the islands who had had measles many years before did not get sick during the epidemic.

Measles was found to be a viral infection in 1911, but the virus was not isolated until 1954.

Before the vaccine, large epidemics occurred every 2 to 3 years, peaking in the late winter and early spring. Measles is highly contagious, and before the vaccine almost everyone got it by 18 years of age. In Canada, about 300,000 to 400,000 cases occurred every year. Nine out of every 10 cases were in children under 10 years old; and more than half were in children 5 to 9 years old.

Children younger than 12 months old and adults were at highest risk of complications and death. Every year in Canada, measles caused several hundred deaths, about 5,000 hospital admissions and 400 cases of encephalitis.

After vaccine

Soon after the measles virus was isolated, ways were found to grow it in tissue culture cells. Measles vaccine was approved for use in 1963. Since then, there has been a dramatic decline in the annual number of measles cases in every country with routine immunization programs.

Remarkable success. In Canada, the number of measles cases fell rapidly after 1963. After a routine two-dose vaccination schedule was introduced in 1996–97, the average number of cases per year fell by more than 99.9% from numbers reported in the decade before vaccine. However, outbreaks still occurred.

There has been a similar decline in measles-related deaths and complications such as encephalitis and SSPE. Before the vaccine, there were 50 to 60 cases of SSPE every year in the United States. With widespread measles immunization, this disease has now become very rare.

Countries with strong vaccination programs have gained remarkable control of measles, with spread of the virus virtually eliminated. Most cases occurring in Canada since 1998 have been "imported", meaning a person became infected outside Canada and developed measles after arriving home from overseas. In recent years, imported measles has led to several outbreaks in Canada, with most cases being children and adolescents who were not fully immunized.

How outbreaks happen

- People travel, contract measles, then bring it home to share.
- In December 2014, an outbreak starting with visitors to Disneyland, California, spread to several other states, to Canada and to Mexico.
- In the Fraser Valley in 2014, 375 cases occurred after a traveller brought measles back from the Netherlands. In 2013, in southern Alberta, a student spread the disease to 42 others after a visit to the Netherlands. In Quebec in 2011, visitors to France brought it back and over 700 persons were infected.
- Where immunization rates are less than 95%, measles spreads very fast.

Unfounded claims. In the late 1990s, a physician in the United Kingdom reported finding a link between measles vaccine and autism. Ever since, large studies by major medical bodies around the world have shown—repeatedly—that there is no relationship between measles vaccine and autism. In 2010, the original report suggesting an association between measles vaccine and autism was found to be fraudulent and was retracted, and the U.K.'s General Medical Council found that the physician had acted "dishonestly and irresponsibly" in doing his research.

Unfortunately, the extensive publicity given to this unfounded allegation has led some parents to refuse the vaccine for their children. In certain countries, measles vaccination rates have decreased and the number of cases of measles has increased.

The germ

Measles virus only infects humans.

How the germ causes illness

When a person inhales droplets containing measles viruses, these germs infect cells lining the nose and throat, then spread to lymph glands in the neck. After multiplying there for 2 to 3 days, the virus enters the bloodstream and spreads to other lymph glands as well as to the liver, spleen and bone marrow, where it grows for another 3 to 5 days. The virus then reinvades the bloodstream and spreads to the skin, eyes, respiratory tract and other organs. The amount of virus in the blood reaches a peak about 11 to 14 days after exposure, then declines rapidly over the next few days.

The measles virus has two proteins in its outer coat that help the virus to attach to human cells and get inside them. Once inside, the virus takes over the cell and makes new viral particles that then infect other cells.

Damages many parts of the body. Measles causes damage to the respiratory tract, lymph glands, spleen, liver, intestines and skin. Damaged cells lining the nose and throat cause a runny nose and sore throat. Damage to the bronchi (airways) makes coughing severe: almost all children with measles have bronchitis. As the virus multiplies in the lymph glands, liver and spleen, inflammation also occurs, causing organ swelling and tenderness. Many infants and young children with measles have diarrhea caused by damage to the intestinal tract.

Affects the immune system. Measles also weakens a person's immune system by affecting the activity of special white blood cells, called lymphocytes. The immune system can't respond nearly as well to other infections for about one month. Measles also lowers the activity of white blood cells responsible for killing bacteria.

Children with measles often get ear infections and pneumonia because of respiratory tract damage and their weaker immunity to bacteria.

How measles virus spreads

Measles virus spreads very easily from person to person. When an infected person coughs or sneezes, droplets containing many virus particles can land in the nose or throat of another person or become airborne (spread through the air).

Also, how measles progresses as an illness virtually guarantees that the virus will spread. Children are highly contagious before the illness is even diagnosed. Most have a runny nose, cough and fever for 2 to 4 days before the typical rash appears. They shed large amounts of virus from the nose, throat and bronchi during this time, and are infectious for a full 8 days: 4 days before and 4 days after the start of the rash.

The illness

Early symptoms (before rash appears). The incubation period for measles, meaning the time between exposure to the virus and the start of symptoms, is about 10 days (with a range of 7 to 18 days).

Symptoms similar to a bad cold precede the rash by 2 to 4 days. They include fever, aches and pains, runny nose, red, inflamed eyes, and cough. The fever increases over the first few days, usually reaching 39.4–40°C by the time rash appears. The cough is frequent and severe. Almost all children with measles have bronchitis (infection of the airways).

During this phase, spots may be seen inside the mouth, usually on the inner cheek opposite the molars. Called "Koplik spots", they are unique to measles and look like small grains of sand on a red base. They disappear 1 to 2 days after the skin rash appears.

Skin rash. Large red spots appear first on the face and head, then spread down over the body to the arms and legs. Spots on the face and upper body can become so large that it looks like there is no normal skin in between them. The rash begins to fade after about a week.

The total illness lasts, on average, 7 to 14 days. The cough lasts longer than any of the other symptoms.

Complications

Complications of measles are common because:
- respiratory tract damage can be extensive, and
- white blood cells, which defend the body against infection, do not function as well.

Measles can cause death, even in previously healthy children. Complications and death happen most often in infants (babies under a year old) and in adults. But even without complications, measles is a severe illness in children. Almost all children have a high fever, severe cough, poor appetite, and are so sick that they must stay in bed for a week or more.

Rate of complications and related deaths. If a child's fever is high for more than 2 days after the rash appears, or if a child's fever comes back, there may be a complicating bacterial infection. Ear infections complicate measles in 7% to 9% of children, bacterial pneumonia occurs in 1% to 6%, and diarrhea in 6%. Infants and children who are poorly nourished or chronically ill have more complications. About 1% of children with measles are hospitalized because of the disease or complications, and death still occurs in about 1 to 2 of every 1,000 cases.

SSPE is another rare but fatal complication of measles (see below).

Measles is especially severe in people whose immune systems have been seriously compromised by disease or medical treatment (e.g., children born with an immunodeficiency or people being treated for cancer).

The most common causes of death are pneumonia and encephalitis (an intense inflammation of the brain).

Pneumonia. Measles always infects the lower respiratory tract, causing bronchitis and cough. Pneumonia develops in 1% to 6% of cases, caused either by the virus itself or by bacteria invading areas damaged by measles. A child whose cough is lingering or getting worse and who is having difficulty breathing may have pneumonia. Treatment for pneumonia includes antibiotics, hospitalization and oxygen if respiratory distress is severe.

Encephalitis occurs in about 1 in every 1,000 cases of measles. Symptoms of encephalitis include fever, seizures and not seeming fully conscious or awake. Many children go into coma. There is no effective treatment for measles encephalitis. About one-third of children with encephalitis die, one-third of survivors have significant permanent brain damage, and one-third recover. It can take a few weeks to many months to recover from encephalitis.

SSPE—rare but fatal. SSPE (subacute sclerosing panencephalitis) is a rare complication of measles, occurring in about 1 or 2 of every 100,000 cases. SSPE is more likely to happen in children who get measles before they are 2 years old. Reports in the 1990s from Canada and the United States suggest that the rate may be as high as 20 per 100,000 cases of measles.

SSPE is caused by chronic infection of brain cells with measles virus. The immune system attacks infected cells and destroys nerve cells in the brain. The illness begins about 7 years after the attack of measles, but may occur earlier. A person with SSPE deteriorates in stages, experiencing: changes in personality and behaviour, intellectual impairment, seizures and coma. There is no cure for SSPE, although some drugs may slow the rate of deterioration. **SSPE is always fatal.**

During pregnancy. Measles infection in pregnancy can be severe, with risks of miscarriage, premature labour or low birth weight in infancy. Unlike rubella, which is sometimes called "German measles", measles does not cause fetal malformation during pregnancy.

Diagnosis

Most parents and physicians in Canada today have never seen a child with measles. However, a child who has a red rash for 3 days or longer, a fever of 38.4°C or higher, and cough, conjunctivitis (pink eye) and a runny nose, might have measles. While these symptoms are more likely to be caused by other viruses, the risk of measles is still present in newcomers to Canada, children and youth who have travelled recently, and other people who may not be fully vaccinated.

Laboratory tests are needed to confirm diagnosis of measles. The virus can be found in saliva during the first few days of illness and specific antibody can be found in a blood sample once the rash has started.

Treatment

There is no specific treatment for measles.

Antibiotics don't treat measles—but may treat complications. Antibiotics are not routinely prescribed to prevent bacterial complications of measles. Studies suggest that the rate of complications from measles is probably the same whether children are treated with antibiotics or not. **Antibiotics are only needed when a bacterial infection complicates measles.**

An **antiviral drug, ribavirin,** has been used to treat children who are severely ill with measles. It is not yet clear how effective this medication is. Ribavirin must be given in hospital.

Large doses of **vitamin A** have been shown to reduce the death rate from measles in infants and young children in developing countries. Children in many poorer countries don't get enough vitamin A. While this treatment may not benefit well-nourished children, vitamin A deficiency has been found in children in the United States and other developed countries. Also, children with severe measles have lower vitamin A levels.

> **Vitamin A may help**
> The World Health Organization recommends that vitamin A be given to *all* children with measles, regardless of where they live.

Post-recovery

Immunity following measles is life-long.

The vaccine

Type of vaccine

Live attenuated virus vaccine. Measles vaccine is a live virus vaccine that has been attenuated (weakened). This means that the vaccine contains a live virus that multiplies in the body after it is given by injection, but it does not cause measles. Rather, it acts like natural infection: the virus infects, multiplies and stimulates immunity.

The vaccine virus does not cause any illness in most people (see "Possible side effects of measles vaccine", below).

How measles vaccine is made

Producing weakened strains. The measles vaccine strains currently used in Canada are known as the "modified Edmonston strain" and the "Schwarz strain". These viruses were weakened by repeatedly growing them in chick embryo tissue culture cells.

Process. The weakened measles virus is grown in chick embryo cell cultures, then extracted and purified. It is combined with mumps and rubella vaccines (as MMR) or with mumps, rubella and varicella vaccines (as MMRV), and freeze-dried.

For general information on vaccine additives, see Chapter 4.

Available forms of measles vaccine

Combinations. Measles vaccine is only available in Canada in combination with mumps and rubella (MMR) or with mumps, rubella and varicella (MMRV) vaccines.

Measles vaccine is given as a single vaccine in many countries in the developing world but is not available this way in Canada. For more information, see "Vaccine types" in Chapter 4.

Vaccines for children, adolescents and adults. The same MMR vaccines and dosage are used for all age groups.

MMRV is not recommended for individuals over 12 years of age because it has not yet been tested in adolescents and adults.

How the vaccine is given

The freeze-dried combination MMR or MMRV vaccine is mixed with sterile distilled water and is usually given as a single injection beneath the skin. The MMRV vaccine and one brand of MMR vaccine may also be injected into muscle.

For more information, see "Getting the shot" in Chapter 4.

Schedule of vaccination

Infants and children (under age 7). Young children in Canada receive 2 doses of MMR or MMRV vaccine. The first dose is at 12 to 15 months of age. The second dose is given at age 18 months in some provinces and territories and later in others. The second dose must be given, at the latest, before school entry (at age 4 to 6 years of age). Both schedules are effective.

Children and adolescents (7 to 17 years of age). Older children and teens *not* previously immunized should get 2 doses of vaccine containing measles.
• MMR or MMRV may be used in children up to 12 years of age.
• Anyone over 12 years old should get MMR.

MMR doses should be *at least* 4 weeks apart and MMRV doses *at least* 6 weeks apart.

Adults born before 1970 are generally presumed to be immune to measles, since they probably had the disease, and are not routinely given the vaccine. **People born in 1970 or since** who are not immune should receive at least one dose of MMR vaccine.

Some adults are more likely than others to come into contact with measles. Health care workers, students, military personnel and travellers to places outside of North America may need extra doses, depending on year of birth.

Boosters (to enhance prior vaccinations). Boosters are usually not needed if someone has received 2 doses of a vaccine containing measles (MMR or MMRV).

Long-lasting protection. Immunity after 2 doses of measles vaccine lasts for many years, if not for life.

Preventing measles after exposure: Post-exposure control

Vaccine

MMR or MMRV can be given to unimmunized or partially immunized people to prevent measles if given within 72 hours of being in contact with a person with measles.

> **Measles is an emergency**
>
> Public Health officials are notified. Exposed non-immune persons are given vaccine or immunoglobulin. People who are unimmunized may be excluded from school or other classroom settings.

Passive immunization: Immune globulin

Immune globulin (IG) is used to prevent or modify measles if vaccine cannot be given. IG is given by injection into muscle. It contains a large amount of antibody against measles virus. Antibodies coat the virus particles, enabling white blood cells to destroy the virus before it can cause any damage.

Does IG work? IG prevents measles in about 80% of exposed people and reduces the severity of illness in most individuals who do become ill. For IG to be effective, the injection must be given as soon as possible after exposure to measles. There is no benefit if more than 6 days have gone by since exposure.

How is IG made? IG is prepared from plasma (the liquid part of blood) from volunteer blood donors, using methods that concentrate the antibodies. A person injected with IG gets a concentrated dose of measles antibody.

Is IG safe? Current methods of testing blood from volunteer donors and of preparing IG ensure that there is no risk of acquiring HIV, hepatitis B, hepatitis C or any other known virus from this product. Other than pain at the injection site, there are almost no significant reactions to IG. Rarely, allergic reactions have been reported.

Who should have IG after exposure to measles?

IG is recommended for non-immune individuals who have been exposed to measles and are at increased risk of severe disease and/ or complications of measles:
- Young infants (under 6 months old)
- Pregnant women who have not had measles or measles vaccine
- People who are immunocompromised.

IG is also recommended for otherwise healthy non-immune individuals over 6 months of age who were in close contact with someone with measles more than 72 hours earlier (i.e., too late to be protected by vaccine).

Possible side effects of measles vaccine

Mild. Side effects after measles vaccine are usually mild after one dose and uncommon after the second dose.

Fever and rash. The most common side effect is fever. Six to 23 days after MMR immunization, about 5% of children have a fever (with or without mild rash) that lasts for 1 to 3 days. This response to vaccine is much less severe than having measles, when 100% of cases experience fever, rash, cough and bronchitis lasting 7 to 14 days. The fever after receiving vaccine is occasionally high enough to cause a seizure in children who are prone to febrile seizures (convulsions caused by fever).

For more information on febrile seizures, see "Vaccine side effects, common and uncommon" and "Side effects of combination vaccines" in Chapter 6.

Other possible side effects. Swollen glands or joint pain occasionally occur after receiving MMR vaccine.

Severe adverse events are rare in healthy children.

A few children (3 or 4 per 100,000 doses of vaccine) develop **thrombocytopenia** (low blood platelets) within 6 weeks of receiving MMR or MMRV vaccine. The decrease in platelets causes small hemorrhages and bruises in the skin. This condition may be caused by the rubella vaccine in MMR.

Measles vaccine may temporarily interfere with skin and **blood tests for tuberculosis**, making the results of these tests unreliable for up to 4 weeks after vaccination.

People with immunosuppression (compromised immune function) should not be given the MMR vaccine. Measles vaccine has, on rare occasions, caused serious diseases such as encephalitis and severe pneumonia when given to individuals whose immune system was severely suppressed by disease or treatment.

Encephalitis (brain inflammation) occurs in about one case per million doses of measles vaccine, but it is not known for sure whether the vaccine causes this condition. Measles disease causes encephalitis in about one of every 1000 cases.

There is no scientific evidence that measles vaccine causes subacute sclerosing panencephalitis (**SSPE**). This brain infection has all but disappeared in countries with effective vaccination programs, while measles disease causes SSPE in at least 1 or 2 of every 100,000 cases.

For more information on possible side effects after receiving the combination vaccines, see Chapter 6, Adverse events and common concerns.

> **Studies show no link to other diseases or disorders**
>
> **Measles vaccine (by itself or combined in the MMR/MMRV vaccines) does not cause autism** or any other kind of brain damage or developmental delay.

Unfounded concerns

Many large, strong scientific studies have looked for serious side effects of measles vaccine and no links have been found (see Chapter 6, Adverse events and common concerns).

People are not infection-prone after vaccination. Some studies report laboratory tests showing that measles vaccine, like measles virus, may lower immune system activity. However, this effect is *much* less pronounced after measles vaccination than after measles infection and, more importantly, is not sufficient to make a person more vulnerable to other infections.

Reasons to avoid or delay measles vaccine

Immunosuppression (compromised immune function). As with all live virus vaccines, measles vaccine is not given to people with a serious immune system disorder caused by disease or certain therapies.

For more information, see Chapter 3, When extra protection is needed.

During pregnancy. Measles vaccine is not given in pregnancy because of a *theoretical risk* of transmitting the vaccine virus to the fetus. But there is *no evidence that measles vaccine can harm the fetus.* Ideally, a woman who needs to be immunized should delay pregnancy by 4 weeks following vaccination with MMR. But if the vaccine was given before she knew she was pregnant, there is no need for concern or for the pregnancy to be terminated.

A pregnant woman's other children should be vaccinated according to the routine schedule. The virus contained in the measles vaccine does not spread from person to person.

Recent injection with IG or other blood products. Immune globulin (IG) and other blood products may contain antibody to measles virus that will interfere with vaccine effectiveness. Vaccination must be delayed for 3 to 11 months, depending on the type and dosage of IG or other blood product used.

Active untreated tuberculosis can be made worse by natural measles infection, but there is no evidence that measles vaccine has the same effect. Nevertheless, measles vaccine is not given to people with untreated active tuberculosis until after their treatment has begun.

For general information on reasons to delay or avoid a vaccine or vaccines, see Chapter 6.

The results of vaccination

Long-lasting protection. Measles vaccine activates a very similar immune response to that caused by measles infection. And although the vaccine virus multiplies in the body, it has never been found in the blood following vaccination, is not excreted from the nose or throat, and cannot spread between people.

After measles vaccine, protective antibodies appear in the blood within 12 days and reach peak concentrations within 21 to 28 days. The amount of antibody activated by the vaccine is lower than after a case of measles, but immunity still lasts for many years after vaccination and may be life-long.

Measles vaccine is not 100% effective. Each dose of measles vaccine is about 95% effective when given on or after a child's first birthday. That means if all 100 children in a school program are vaccinated, 5 will still be non-immune to measles after one dose.

Not all children get vaccinated. Only one child with measles in a school where 5 of 100 children are non-immune is a serious health risk.

Measles is highly contagious. The infection will probably spread to all 5 non-immune children—even though they have received one dose of vaccine.

> **Measles vaccine: Why 2 doses are needed**
> Long after the start of routine vaccination in 1963, measles cases were still occurring in Canada, even in vaccinated children when outbreaks occurred in schools.

The current two-dose schedule works much better. In countries with strong vaccination programs, children are given one dose of measles vaccine in infancy and a second dose before starting school.

The second dose ensures that the number of non-immune children is extremely low.

Vaccine failure—reasons and remedies

Maternal antibody. About 5% to 10% of infants don't respond to their first dose of measles vaccine. There are a number of reasons why, the most important being that a mother transfers protective antibodies to her baby near the end of pregnancy. If maternal antibodies are still present when the first dose of vaccine is given, the vaccine virus may be inactivated before it can stimulate the infant's immune system.

Antibodies from the mother disappear over time, usually before one year of age. In a few children, maternal antibodies may last longer, preventing an immune response to the first dose of vaccine.

Vaccine success

Evidence that measles vaccine works:
- The number of measles cases per year dropped dramatically (by 99.9%) after the routine two-dose vaccination schedule was introduced in Canada in 1996–97.
- In the United Kingdom, where unsubstantiated fears that measles vaccine caused autism were strongest, parents now have a renewed appreciation of measles risks and vaccine safety. Immunization rates fell from over 93% to less than 85% after 2000, causing serious outbreaks in England, Scotland and Ireland. Fortunately, measles vaccination rates are now on the increase.
- **Mass campaigns.** In 1996, a mass vaccination program was started in Ontario and Quebec. All school-children were vaccinated and school outbreaks were brought under control.
- Eradicating measles worldwide is realistic. Measles vaccination programs have been so successful that the World Health Organization is now working by to eliminate the disease from the world by 2020. Eradicating measles in developing countries is a challenge because so many unvaccinated children also live with conditions that reinforce disease: overcrowding, poverty and inadequate health care.

Snapshots

- Measles is not "a mild infection that all children should have". Measles was, and is, a severe illness with a high rate of complications and a real risk of permanent disability and death.
- Measles-containing vaccines are very safe and provide the same protection against measles that the natural illness provides— without the risk of severe illness or complications.
- All children should be vaccinated against measles unless they have a serious disorder of the immune system caused by disease or certain treatments.
- Measles vaccine, alone or combined in the MMR or MMRV vaccine, does not cause autism, or any other kind of brain damage or developmental delay.

- Two doses of measles vaccine are needed because about 5% of vaccinated children remain unprotected following their first dose.
- Because measles is so contagious, populations with even a small number of unimmunized or inadequately immunized people remain at risk of measles outbreaks.
- There are obstacles to overcome before global measles vaccination programs can be completely successful. But with perseverance and time, it is possible to eradicate measles completely from the world.

15

Meningococcal disease

The bacterium called meningococcus (or *Neisseria meningitidis*) causes bacteremia, septicemia, meningitis and other invasive infections.

- Meningitis is an infection of the membranes and fluid that cover the brain and spinal cord.
- Bacteremia is an infection of the bloodstream
- Severe bacteremia is called septicemia. It can progress rapidly, causing shock (a sudden drop in blood pressure) and damage to many organs in the body. If untreated, overwhelming shock can cause death.

Even with treatment and intensive care, severe meningococcal disease can kill.

There are 13 different types of meningococci, which are distinguished by differences in the bacteria's outer coating. Groups A, B, C, Y and W135 cause almost all cases of meningococcal disease. There can be many different strains in each group.

A history of meningococcal disease

Before vaccine

Before 1950, group A strains caused very large epidemics every 7 to 10 years in many parts of the world. The last such epidemic in Canada was between 1940 and 1943, with more than 3000 cases. Fortunately, no large group A epidemics have occurred in Canada, the United States or other developed nations since the end of World War II.

Very large epidemics of group A disease continue to occur in other parts of the world: almost every year in the "meningitis belt" (sub-Saharan Africa), and less frequently in China, India, and other countries with limited resources.

Since 1950, group B and group C strains have caused most cases of meningococcal disease in Canada.

After vaccine

The United States army developed effective vaccines against groups A and C meningococci in the late 1960s. Meningococcal outbreaks had always been a problem in the military, especially among recruits in wartime. The group C vaccine was almost 90% effective in preventing disease in army recruits between 1968 and 1970. Since 1972, military recruits in the United States, Canada and many other countries have been routinely vaccinated, and group C outbreaks in the armed forces have disappeared.

Groups A and C vaccines (individually and combined) have been effective in controlling outbreaks of disease, both in the general population and among military recruits.

Unfortunately, the original group C vaccine was not effective in children under 2 years old, the group most at risk for disease. Also, early meningococcal vaccines did not protect people longer than 3 to 5 years, so they were not useful for routine immunization.

Fortunately, as with Hib and pneumococcal vaccines (see Chapters 9 and 18), a conjugate form of the vaccine was developed that is very effective in protecting infants (children under 12 months of age), older children and adults.

The meningococcal conjugate vaccine against group C was approved for use in Canada in 2001 and is now given to all infants as part of their routine schedule. Since 2001, the number of cases of group C disease in Canada has dropped by 85%.

While the conjugate vaccine was effective in controlling infections cause by group C strains, the numbers of infections caused by other serotypes didn't change. Group B now causes over 60% of meningococcal infections, with group Y as the second-most frequent cause, at 17%.

A newer form of conjugate vaccine that is effective against group C and also serogroups A, Y and W135 was approved for use in the United States in 2005 and in Canada in 2006. Many provinces and territories now routinely give one dose of this vaccine to adolescents. It is also being used for people of all ages who are at higher risk of meningococcal infection (see Table 15.1).

A vaccine against group B meningococcus was licensed in Canada in 2013. It is not used routinely, but may be given to people at high risk for meningococcal disease and to control outbreaks.

The germ

Meningococcal bacteria infect only humans. Infection always starts in the nose or throat, where the bacteria attach to cells on the surface of the respiratory tract.

Healthy carriage. Most people have no symptoms of illness after being infected with meningococci. They become "carriers" of a "silent" infection in their nose or throat. Most healthy carriers are adolescents and young adults. Few infants are carriers of meningoccoci, and not many children.

> ### Carriage without infection may produce immunity
>
> Meningococci can live in the nose and throat for 6 months or more. Carriage causes an immune response against the specific strain being carried, not against other meningococcal strains. As a person becomes immune to one strain, a new strain can infect the nose and throat and the process of building immunity to the new strain begins.

It is not known why one person becomes a silent carrier while another develops severe disease. But people with certain medical conditions are more likely to become very ill (see Table 15.1).

How the germ causes illness

Infection and illness. Meningococcal bacteria have an external coat, or capsule, made of large, complex sugars (polysaccharides). This capsule protects the bacteria against attack by white blood cells, our body's main defense against infection. If a person doesn't have antibodies to the specific strain of meningococci in their nose and throat, white blood cells can't attack and kill the bacteria. Meningococci then invade the body, multiply freely and cause disease.

While the capsule protects meningococcal bacteria from attack by white blood cells, another part of the wall of the bacteria, called **endotoxin**, causes the damage. When endotoxin is released in the body, it causes an intense reaction called **inflammation**. If the bacterial infection is not treated, inflammation can get out of control and cause damage throughout the body, especially to blood vessels.

How meningococci spread

The spread of meningococci usually involves carriers, but people with meningococcal disease also spread the infection. Carriers can be infected for short periods (weeks) or many months. Cigarette smoking, both active and passive (inhaling second-hand smoke), increases the risk of carriage and, therefore, the risk of spreading the bacteria to others.

Spread from an infected person (carriers included) requires close contact (e.g., kissing or uncovered coughs or sneezes when other people are nearby). The bacteria also spread through saliva when sharing items that have been in the mouth, such as food or drink (e.g., from cutlery, a water bottle, soda can or drinking straws), a lipstick, mouthguard or musical instrument with a mouthpiece.

Not highly contagious

Fortunately, meningococci bacteria are extremely fragile outside the body and do not survive on objects or surfaces. Meningococcal infections are serious but not highly contagious.

Daily contact. The risk of spread increases greatly with daily contact. Family members or other people living with someone who is ill with a meningococcal infection are more at risk. But while the risk of spread within a household is higher than in the general public, it is still comparatively small: illness in other family members only occurs 1% to 3% of the time, and usually within a week of the first person becoming ill.

The illness

Invasive infection. Invasive meningococcal disease most often results in septicemia or meningitis, or both.

Septicemia is the most severe form of meningococcal disease. With this type of infection, bacteria multiply rapidly in the blood and overwhelm the body. They also release endotoxin (poison) from their cell walls. Too much endotoxin causes an intense overreaction by the body's defense system. Chemicals are released that damage small blood vessels and cells in many organs. Normally, these same chemicals help to fight infection but with septicemia, concentrations are far too high. Septicemia can cause shock (a sudden drop in blood pressure) and organ failure.

> ### Meningococcal septicemia is sudden and severe
> The total time from the first symptom of fever to death can be as short as 6 to 12 hours.

Meningitis is caused by bacteria in the blood spreading into the central nervous system. Inflammation and blocked blood vessels can affect blood supply to the brain. Brain cells cannot survive interruption of their blood supply for very long, and inflammation can cause permanent brain damage.

Infection of other body parts. Once meningococci enter the blood-stream, they can infect almost any other part of the body, such as the lungs, joints, bones, heart and skin.

Symptoms of meningococcal disease. A **rash** is the most distinctive symptom of invasive meningococcal disease.

The rash occurs in almost all cases of meningococcal septicemia and in about two-thirds of cases of meningococcal meningitis. Sometimes it does not develop until the disease is quite advanced. The rash is caused by damage to small blood vessels in the skin, which bleed into surrounding tissue. The spots are called *petechiae*.

> ### A distinctive rash
> The rash can start as small red spots anywhere on the body. At first, it may fade when pressed, but within an hour or two, spots no longer fade. The rash may spread all over the body. In severe cases, spots enlarge so rapidly they look like large bruises under the skin.

The early signs of meningococcal septicemia and meningitis can be very similar to those of influenza and other viral infections. This makes diagnosis difficult.

Meningococcal septicemia and meningitis have different symptoms.
Septicemia often begins with fever, aches and pains, nausea, loss of appetite and feeling generally unwell. The rash usually starts within a few hours of the start of the fever and the disease progresses rapidly to shock.

A person with meningitis usually has vomiting, severe headache, and a stiff neck or pain when flexing the neck and back. Sometimes septicemia and meningitis happen together.

Meningitis is difficult to diagnose in infants because some symptoms (e.g., the stiff neck, neck pain, headache) can't be seen. In young infants, the soft spot on the top of the skull may bulge, but this sign usually occurs late in the illness.

Symptoms and signs of meningococcal meningitis in infants

- Fever
- Fretfulness or irritability, especially when handled
- Difficulty waking
- Difficulty feeding
- Vomiting
- Bulging of the fontanelle
- Rash that does not go away when you press on the spots

Infection in other body parts. Symptoms of infection in other parts of the body are specific to the part affected. For example, with arthritis, there is pain in the joint or bone.

Complications

Invasive meningococcal diseases can be rapid and severe. About 7% of cases will die, in spite of prompt diagnosis and appropriate treatment.

Deafness occurs in 1% to 2% of survivors of meningitis. Permanent brain damage is uncommon.

Gangrene (destruction of skin, muscles and other tissues) caused by meningococcal septicemia can cause permanent scarring and sometimes leads to amputation.

Kidney damage can also occur.

Diagnosis

The distinctive rash may help with diagnosis. Unlike most rashes caused by an allergy or viral infection, the meningococcal rash does not fade under pressure. When the side of a clear glass is pressed against the skin and the rash is examined through it, the rash remains visible. This is known as the "tumbler test". In early stages of illness, when the rash first appears, it may fade under pressure, but as it develops (within a few hours) it no longer fades. Spots may converge into large areas that look like bruising and turn dark red, but not all children with meningococccal infection develop this type of rash.

Tests are needed. Diagnosing meningococcal disease depends on finding the bacteria in blood or cerebrospinal fluid, and sometimes in the skin rash. Cerebrospinal fluid is obtained by inserting a small needle into the spinal canal in the lower back and removing a sample. This fluid is examined in the laboratory for bacteria and for signs of inflammation (white blood cells and changes in concentrations of protein and sugar).

Treatment

Antibiotics. Before antibiotics, meningococcal meningitis and septicemia were almost always fatal. With appropriate medical treatment, the death rate has been reduced to about 10%.

Treatment for septicemia. Patients with septicemia almost always require treatment in an intensive care unit, medications to treat shock and, often, mechanical ventilation to help with breathing.

Family members. When one case of serious meningococcal disease occurs in a family, there is a risk that the bacteria have already spread to others in the household. To prevent illness, all family or household members are given an antibiotic to clear the bacteria from the nose and throat. They may be given vaccine as well.

Post-recovery

Immunity that develops after a meningococcal infection is directed mainly against the specific strain that caused disease and may not protect against other strains in the same group. Vaccination after recovery from any form of meningococcal infection is advised.

The vaccine

Types of vaccines

Purified bacterial polysaccharide. There are two types of meningococcal vaccines, both made from purified complex sugars extracted from the bacteria. Because the vaccines are highly purified extracts and do not contain whole bacteria, it is impossible to get the disease or symptoms of the disease from the vaccine.

Meningococcal polysaccharide vaccines containing substances from groups A, A and C, or A, C, Y and W135, were used in the past in Canada and are still being used in some parts of the world. These vaccines are not used routinely in Canada today because the newer conjugate vaccines work much better.

Meningococcal conjugate vaccine. Group C meningococcal conjugate vaccines were approved for use in Canada in 2001. Like the Hib type b and pneumococcal conjugate vaccines (see Chapters 9 and 18), meningococcal conjugates are made from the purified group C polysaccharide, which is then chemically linked to a purified protein. (Conjugate means "joined together".)

Linking the purified polysaccharide to a protein carrier creates vaccines that are effective in infants as young as 2 months old.

A combined conjugate containing vaccines against groups A, C, Y and W135 was approved for use in the United States in 2005 and in Canada in 2006. This vaccine protects against all four groups of meningococcus.

A new vaccine against group B meningococcus was licensed in Canada in 2013. Unlike the other meningocooccal vaccines, it does not contain polysaccharide. The polysaccharide from group B meningococcus can't be used to make vaccine because it does not stimulate an immune response. Instead, proteins from the surface of group B meningoococcus are used. As with the polysaccharide vaccines, these proteins are highly purified chemicals, not intact bacteria, so it is impossible to get the disease (or symptoms of the disease) from the vaccine.

So far, this vaccine is recommended routinely only for people at high risk of meningococcal disease. It can be used in children who are 2 months of age or older.

How meningococcal vaccines are made

Process for meningococcal conjugate vaccines. First, the bacteria are grown in liquid culture. When growth is complete, the bacteria are removed and the polysaccharide is extracted and purified. The purified polysaccharide is then chemically linked to a highly purified protein (tetanus toxoid or CRM, a protein similar to diphtheria toxoid).

Process for the meningococcal A, C, Y and W135 conjugate vaccine. Each type of bacteria is grown separately. The same process as above is followed to produce the four conjugates, using diphtheria or tetanus toxoid or CRM. The four conjugates are then combined to make the final product.

Process for meningococcal group B vaccine. The four proteins contained in this vaccine are found just under the capsule of many, but not all, meningococcal B strains. One component is created by growing meningococcus B in liquid culture as above, then purifying the protein. Other components are produced by molecular technology using nucleic acids (genes) isolated from the group B meningococcus. These components are then combined in one vaccine.

For general information on vaccine additives, see Chapter 4.

Available forms of meningococcal vaccine

Three meningococcal **group C** conjugate vaccines are available in Canada from different manufacturers. The vaccines differ in the protein used to make the conjugate.

As of 2014, there are three vaccines containing conjugates against **groups A, C, Y and W135.** These also differ in the protein conjugates used.

There is only one meningococcal vaccine for group B.

None of the meningococcal vaccines licensed in Canada are available in combination with any other vaccine.

Vaccines for different age groups. Meningococcal vaccines for various age groups do not differ, except that only one form of the A-C-Y-W135 conjugate vaccine is currently recommended for use in children as young as 2 months old.

All vaccines work equally well in the age groups for which they are recommended.

How the vaccines are given

All the vaccines against meningococcus are given by injection into muscle. For more information, see "Getting the shot" in Chapter 4.

Schedules of vaccination

Meningococcal conjugate vaccines. As of 2014, all provinces and territories in Canada provide one routine dose of meningococcal conjugate C vaccine at 12 months of age. Some also provide earlier doses, starting at 2 months of age. Children younger than 5 years old who have not been immunized should also receive one dose, and the vaccine may also be considered for older unvaccinated children.

All provinces and territories also provide a routine dose of either meningococcal conjugate C or A-C-Y-W135 during adolescence.

All children at high risk of meningococcal disease (see Table 15.1) should receive one or more doses of **meningococcal A-C-Y-W135 conjugate** vaccine starting at 2 months of age. The number of doses depends on a child's age, diagnosis and the type of vaccine that is chosen.

As of 2014, no province or territory in Canada is routinely providing the meningococcal group B vaccine. However, it can be given as to children as young as 2 months old and is recommended for individuals at high risk of disease and for close contacts of people with group B disease. It is also recommended during outbreaks of group B disease. The number of doses to be given depends on age.

Boosters (to enhance prior vaccinations). Other than the dose given in adolescence, booster doses are not routinely recommended.

Boosters are recommended for persons at risk for meningococcal disease (see Table 15.1) and for all close contacts of someone with invasive meningococcal disease. Boosters of conjugate vaccine are given after 3 to 5 years to children younger than 6 years old, and every 5 years in older people. Boosters are given earlier to the household contacts of a person with meningococcal disease.

It is not yet known whether booster doses will be required for the new meningococcus B vaccine.

Length of protection. Protection following immunization with the meningococcal C conjugate vaccine decreases with time and how long protection actually lasts is not known. Because there is now almost no group C disease in Canada, a booster is routinely given only in adolescence. However, as noted above, people at high risk of meningococcal disease are given boosters.

The protective effects of meningococcal A-C-Y-W135 conjugate vaccine may start to decrease 3 years after the vaccine is given. However, routine booster doses are currently not recommended in Canada for healthy adolescents because meningococcal disease is rare in this age group at the present time.

We do not yet know how long protection lasts following immunization with the meningococcal B conjugate vaccine.

Table 15.1
People at higher risk of invasive meningococcal disease

Individuals with certain disorders of the immune system
• Sickle cell disease and certain other congenital disorders of hemoglobin (red blood cells)
• Absent spleen or a spleen that does not work well because of a congenital defect, disease or surgery
• Inability or reduced ability to make antibodies
• Deficiency of the complement system (a part of the immune system that defends against meningococcus) or taking medications that affect the complement system
• HIV infection

Individuals at risk of exposure to meningococcus
• Household contacts of someone with invasive meningococcal infection
• Travellers to areas of the world where meningococcal infection is common
• Persons who work with meningococcus in a laboratory
• The military

For more information see Chapter 3, When extra protection is needed.

Possible side effects of meningococcal vaccines

Both the C and the A-C-Y-W135 meningococcal conjugate vaccines are very safe. Both have been given to millions of children.

Local reactions (e.g., redness, swelling, tenderness) occur at the site of the injection in 10% to 50% of people who get this shot, but the reactions are mild and last only 1 to 2 days.

Fever, irritability and other general reactions are *not* more frequent or severe when the meningococcal conjugate vaccine is given at the same time as any of the combination vaccines (for infants) or with hepatitis B vaccine (for school children).

The meningococcal group B vaccine is much newer. Experience so far indicates that it is safe, but fever is very common. Infants who are given this vaccine at the same visit as other routine vaccines have more fever.

Reasons to delay or avoid meningococcal vaccine

For general information on reasons to delay or avoid a vaccine or vaccines, see Chapter 6.

The results of vaccination

Evidence that meningococcal vaccines work:
- Group A and group C polysaccharide vaccines have been effective in preventing disease during outbreaks.
- Outbreaks of meningococcal disease among military recruits have been eliminated by routine vaccination with group A-C-Y-W135 polysaccharide vaccine at the start of training.
- Meningococcal conjugate vaccines are effective in protecting against group C disease, and protection against group C strains is largely achieved. In Canada the numbers of cases of meningococcal C disease in all age groups has decreased by 84% with routine immunization.

Snapshots

- Meningococcal vaccines are very safe and effective.
- The routine immunization of infants with the group C conjugate vaccine is very effective in preventing group C disease.
- Recently introduced vaccination programs for boosters in adolescence are expected to reduce further the number of cases of meningococcal disease that occur in Canada each year.
- It is too early to know if routine use of group A, C, Y and W135 vaccine in adolescents in some Canadian provinces and territories has decreased the incidence of meningococcal disease in this age group.
- The next step in controlling meningococcal disease would be routine use of an effective vaccine against group B.
- It is too early to know the effectiveness of the group B vaccine that was recently licensed in Canada.

16

Mumps

Mumps is an infection caused by a virus. Typical symptoms include fever, headache and swelling of the salivary glands around the jaw and cheeks. About 1 in 10 people also get mumps meningitis, an infection of the fluid and lining that cover the brain and spinal cord. Usually, mumps meningitis is mild and does not cause permanent harm.

Mumps can also cause encephalitis, an intense inflammation of the brain, which can lead to permanent brain damage. Other complications of mumps include deafness, a painful swelling of the testicles in teenage boys and men, and painful infection of the ovaries in women. In rare cases, men with both testicles infected with mumps become sterile.

A history of mumps

Before vaccine

Before vaccination began in the early 1970s, mumps was very common in Canada, with at least 30,000 cases reported each year. This number doesn't include cases unreported by doctors or mild cases never seen by a doctor, meaning the annual total was much higher. Before the vaccine, mumps was the most common cause of encephalitis (inflammation of the brain) in children, and a common cause of deafness. Children under 15 years old had 90% of all infections, and infections were most common in 5- to 9- year-olds.

After vaccine

Where effective vaccination programs are in place:
- The number of mumps cases drops dramatically (by over 90% according to data from Canada, the United States and several European countries).
- Mumps encephalitis almost disappears.

After children in Canada starting receiving 2 doses of the measles-mumps-rubella (MMR) vaccine in 1996–97, reported cases of mumps dropped by 99.8% compared with before the vaccine was introduced.

However, a few large mumps outbreaks have occurred in Canada since 2006, mostly affecting young adults who received only one dose of mumps vaccine as children. These individuals are more vulnerable than people

Outbreaks happen

In 2007–08, a large mumps outbreak started in Nova Scotia and spread to other provinces, mainly affecting 20- to 29-year-olds in post-secondary educational settings. This prompted the recommendation for a second dose of mumps vaccine for both students and staff in high schools, colleges and universities.

born before 1970, who have often had the disease and are immune, or children who have received 2 doses and are more completely immunized. In every outbreak, the initial mumps cases were imported from elsewhere but then spread locally.

The germ

Mumps virus only infects humans.

How the germ causes illness

Mumps starts as an infection of the nose and throat, and often spreads to the salivary glands located at the angle of the jaw. Once the virus enters the bloodstream it can infect many other body parts: the brain, the covering of the brain and spinal cord, the testicles or ovaries, the pancreas, kidneys, breasts, thyroid, joints or the inner ear.

How mumps spreads

Spread of mumps virus requires close contact between people. An infected person's cough or sneeze spreads droplets containing many virus particles to the nose or throat of another person. Mumps virus also spreads through contact with saliva (e.g., by kissing, or sharing a mouthed toy, food or drinks).

Close contact
In Canada since 2000, more adolescents and young adults have contracted mumps from close contact at bars, dances and other social events than by sharing college dorm rooms.

A fairly long contagious period. People with mumps are contagious from about 7 days before salivary glands start to swell until up to 5 days afterward. Many children (almost 60%) and some adults infected with mumps do not develop swollen glands or other significant symptoms, but they can still spread the virus.

Mumps is **less contagious than measles or chickenpox**. Studies show that only one-third of non-immune family members get mumps following illness in a child.

> **Mild illness is still contagious**
> - About 20% of children with mumps have no symptoms of illness.
> - Another 40% have a minor illness like a cold, and are not recognized to have mumps.
> - Some adults infected with mumps do not have typical symptoms.
>
> But all these groups can still spread the virus to others.

The illness

Symptoms. The incubation period for mumps, meaning the time between exposure to the virus and the start of symptoms, is longer than that for measles or chickenpox. Illness develops an average of 16 to 18 days after exposure.

About half of cases with symptoms have a minor illness similar to a cold, and half get swollen salivary glands ("typical" mumps is described below).

Children under 2 years old and older adults are more likely than preschool and young school-age children to have mild infections without swollen salivary glands. Mumps is more severe and complications are more frequent in young adults.

"Typical" or classic mumps usually starts with fever, aches and pains, and loss of appetite. After one or more days, the salivary glands begin to swell and feel tender. Chewing and swallowing become painful. The parotid glands (the largest of the salivary glands, located in front of the ear and behind the angle of the jaw) often swell. Both sides of the face are enlarged in about half of cases. Other salivary glands are affected in 30% to 40% of cases.

Other symptoms in children and adolescents may include fever, headache, neck stiffness, stomach ache and drowsiness, confusion or dizziness.

Length of illness. When mumps was a common illness, it usually lasted for quite a while: fever for 3 days; pain, 5 days; swelling, 8 days; and 3 days in bed. People missed about 7 days of work or school. Most were back to normal within 14 days.

Complications

Mumps meningitis, the most common complication, is caused when the virus invades the membranes and fluid covering the brain and spinal cord. Most cases are very mild, and symptoms such as headache, a stiff neck and drowsiness last only a few days. Mumps meningitis occurs in about 5% of cases, is rarely severe, and almost never causes permanent harm.

Mumps encephalitis (inflammation of the brain) is caused by an aggressive reaction of the body to mumps infection. Mumps encephalitis is now extremely rare in Canada but is more likely to occur in adolescents and adults than in children. It can cause permanent brain damage and lead to problems such as recurrent seizures, paralysis or hydrocephalus (too much fluid on the brain).

Infection with mumps virus can damage the auditory nerve and/or inner ear and cause **deafness** in children and adolescents. It is estimated to occur in 0.5 to 5 out of every 100,000 cases. There may no other signs of brain infection, such as meningitis or encephalitis.

Mumps infection causes **pancreatitis** (inflammation of the pancreas) in about 4% of cases, with vomiting and abdominal pain. An association between mumps pancreatitis and diabetes has been suggested but not proven.

In older boys and men. Mumps infection of the testicles (called orchitis) is rare before puberty, but can affect about 20% to 40% of adolescent and adult males with the disease. Most orchitis cases, which can be very painful, involve only one testicle and recovery is complete. Sterility after mumps orchitis is rare even when both testicles are infected but reproductive capacity is lowered in about 13% of cases.

In women. An adult woman with mumps may have painful swelling of the breasts, or abdominal or pelvic pain caused by inflammation of the ovaries (called oophoritis). There is no proof that mumps causes female infertility (an inability to get pregnant).

During pregnancy. Infection with mumps during pregnancy does not affect development of the fetus. As with any infection during pregnancy, a severe illness can result in miscarriage.

Diagnosis

Clinical examination. Diagnosing typical mumps is usually based on swelling of the parotid glands. But many other viruses (such as influenza, parainfluenza, Epstein-Barr and adenovirus) can cause an illness identical to mumps. When there is no mumps outbreak, less than 20% of cases of parotid swelling are due to mumps virus. Also, many people with mumps infection do not have parotid swelling.

A clinical test to find the mumps virus in a sample of saliva, urine or other body fluid may be needed to confirm diagnosis. Tests to detect increases in the amount of mumps antibody in the blood were used in the past but are rarely used now.

Treatment

For symptoms only. There is no effective treatment for mumps. Giving acetaminophen (e.g., Tempra, Tylenol) can reduce pain, and applying a hot or cold compress can ease painful salivary glands. Pain from orchitis can be eased with medication and by elevating the scrotum.

Post-recovery

It is possible to be reinfected with mumps, although it rarely happens. Most recurrent "mumps" cases turn out to be illnesses caused by other viruses. People infected with mumps virus, whether their glands swell or not, almost always develop lifelong immunity to the disease.

The vaccine

Type of vaccine

Live attenuated virus vaccine. Mumps vaccine is a live virus vaccine that has been attenuated (weakened). This means that the vaccine contains a live virus that multiplies in the body after it is given by injection, but it does not cause mumps. Rather, it acts like natural infection: the virus infects, multiplies and stimulates immunity.

The vaccine virus does not cause any illness in most people (see "Possible side effects of mumps vaccine", below).

How mumps vaccine is made

Producing weakened strains. The mumps virus is weakened by repeated growth in hens' eggs, and then in chick embryo cell cultures. A weakened virus vaccine must be able to stimulate immunity without causing illness. Once the weakened strain has been isolated, large amounts of it are grown and stored for future use.

The vaccine strain now used in Canada and the United States is called the "Jeryl Lynn strain", after the child from whom it was first isolated. Nine other vaccine strains have been developed and are used in other countries.

Process. The weakened mumps virus is grown in chick embryo cell cultures, then extracted and purified. It is combined with measles and rubella vaccines (as MMR) or with measles, rubella and varicella vaccines (as MMRV vaccine), and freeze-dried.

For general information on vaccine additives, see Chapter 4.

Available forms of mumps vaccine

Combinations. Mumps vaccine is only available in Canada in combination with measles and rubella (MMR) or with measles, rubella and varicella (MMRV) vaccines. It is not available as a single vaccine in Canada.

Vaccines for children, adolescents and adults. The same MMR vaccines and dosage are used for all age groups.

MMRV is not recommended for individuals over 12 years of age because it has not yet been tested in adolescents and adults.

How the vaccine is given

The freeze-dried combination MMR or MMRV vaccine is mixed with sterile distilled water and is usually given as a single injection beneath the skin. The MMRV vaccine and one brand of MMR vaccine may also be injected into muscle.

For more information, see "Getting the shot", in Chapter 4.

Schedule of vaccination

Infants and children (under age 7). Young children in Canada receive 2 doses of MMR or MMRV vaccine. The first dose is at 12 to 15 months of age. The second is at age 18 months in some provinces and territories and later in others. The second dose must be given, at the latest, before school entry (4 to 6 years of age). Both schedules are effective.

Children and adolescents (7 to 17 years of age). Older children and teens *not* previously immunized should get 2 doses of a vaccine containing mumps:
- MMR or MMRV may be used in children up to 12 years of age.
- Anyone over 12 years old should get MMR.

MMR doses should be at least 4 weeks apart, and MMRV doses *at least* 6 weeks apart.

People born in 1970 or since who are not immune should get at least one dose of MMR vaccine. **Adults born before 1970** are generally presumed to be immune to mumps since they probably had the disease, and are not *routinely* given the vaccine.

Adult students and non-immune travellers to places outside North America need one dose of MMR vaccine if they were born before 1970, and 2 doses if born in 1970 or later. Non-immune health care workers and military personnel need 2 doses regardless of age.

Boosters (to enhance prior vaccinations). Unless there is a mumps outbreak, boosters are usually not needed if someone has received 2 doses of a vaccine containing mumps (MMR or MMRV).

Length of protection. After 2 doses of vaccine, protection lasts many years. However, recent outbreaks of mumps among college students in the United States suggest that immunity after vaccination may wane after 10 to 15 years.

Possible side effects of mumps vaccine

Rare. Side effects of the strain of mumps vaccine now used in Canada have been rare. A few children develop mild swelling of the salivary glands 10 to 14 days after vaccination. Meningitis has been reported to occur at a rate of less than one case per million doses of vaccine, and has no long-term complications. As noted above, meningitis is very common with mumps infection.

Mild meningitis was 10 times more common with a form of mumps vaccine used in the past but not used in Canada in recent decades. No permanent brain damage occurred.

For information on possible side effects after receiving MMR or MMRV vaccine, see Chapter 6, Adverse events and common concerns.

Reasons to avoid or delay mumps vaccine

Immunosuppression (compromised immune system function). As with all live virus vaccines, mumps vaccine is not given to people with a serious immune system disorder caused by disease or certain medications.

For more information, see Chapter 3, When extra protection is needed.

During pregnancy. Mumps vaccine is not given in pregnancy because of a *theoretical risk* of transmitting the vaccine virus to the fetus. But there is *no evidence that mumps vaccine can harm the fetus*. Ideally, a woman who needs to be immunized should delay pregnancy by 4 weeks following vaccination with MMR. But if the vaccine was given before she knew she was pregnant, there is no need for concern or for the pregnancy to be terminated.

A pregnant woman's other children should be vaccinated according to the routine schedule. The virus contained in the mumps vaccine does not spread from person to person.

Recent injection with immune globulin (IG) or other blood products. IG and other blood products may contain antibody to mumps virus that will interfere with vaccine effectiveness. Vaccination must be delayed for 3 to 11 months, depending on the type and dosage of IG or other blood product used.

For general information on reasons to delay or avoid a vaccine or vaccines, see Chapter 6.

The results of vaccination

Evidence that mumps vaccine works:
- Controlled studies have shown that a single dose of mumps vaccine is over 90% effective in preventing mumps.
- After the two-dose MMR vaccination schedule was introduced throughout Canada in 1998, there was a 99.8% decline in the number of mumps cases.
- In Canada, outbreaks have occurred in young adults, who have often received only one dose of vaccine.
- In the United States, outbreaks have occurred recently among young adults who received 2 doses of vaccine as young children, including an outbreak among National Hockey League players in the winter of 2014. These outbreaks may reflect loss of immunity in a population with low overall immunization rates.

- Notably, no outbreaks have occurred in Finland, which has had very high rates of mumps immunization (over 95%) for several decades. Immunization rates are lower in Canada and the United States.

Snapshots

- Mumps is usually a mild infection. Complications are relatively frequent but also, usually, mild. In rare cases, mumps can cause permanent brain damage or deafness, and impair fertility in men.
- Mumps vaccine is very safe and effective.
- All children need to be vaccinated against mumps, as do adolescents and young adults who have not had the disease.
- There is some concern about how long protection lasts after vaccination. The immunity induced by the mumps vaccine does not last as long as immunity after natural mumps infection, and outbreaks still occur.
- Mumps outbreaks usually happen in young adults on college or university campuses, where people of similar ages live close together. People who have had only one dose of vaccine are especially vulnerable. Weakening immunity after vaccine is given in early childhood may also play a role.

17

Pertussis

Pertussis is a respiratory infection caused by bacteria called *Bordetella pertussis*. Pertussis is also known as "whooping cough" because its main symptom is severe spells of coughing followed by a "whoop" sound before the next breath. The illness lasts many weeks. It is sometimes called the "hundred day cough".

A history of pertussis

Before vaccine

Pertussis used to kill many children. In the early 1900s, 5 out of every 1,000 children born in the United States and Canada died of pertussis before reaching their fifth birthday. Before routine vaccination against pertussis, there were between 30,000 and 50,000 cases every year in

Canada, with 50 to 100 deaths. Most deaths involved infants (babies younger than 12 months old).

Infant deaths from pertussis declined by more than 70% between 1900 and 1940 in Canada, the United States and England, thanks in part to less overcrowding and smaller families. But while societal changes reduced the risk of young infants being exposed to pertussis, almost 100% of children still had the infection by the time they were 10 to 12 years of age.

The number of children getting pertussis didn't decrease until there was a vaccine.

After vaccine

After the introduction of whole-cell pertussis vaccine in 1943, the death rate declined even farther and fewer children got the disease.

This form of vaccine contained whole killed pertussis bacteria. And while it was effective, it caused high fever in young infants and painful local reactions. An acellular pertussis vaccine was then developed, using selected purified bacterial proteins instead of whole bacterial cells. This vaccine was better tolerated by infants, more acceptable to parents, and replaced the whole-cell vaccine in Canada in 1997–98.

The routine immunization of infants with acellular pertussis vaccine led to a steady decline in the rate of pertussis among children 6 months to 10 years of age. But the proportion of cases in adolescents and adults has been increasing in Canada since the mid-1990s.

In 1999–2000, Canada added a booster dose of acellular pertussis for adolescents (14 to 16 years old), and rates of the illness continued to decrease. Yet between 2001 and 2011, there were still 1,000 to 3,000 pertussis cases reported each year, mostly in adolescents and young adults.

Outbreaks continue to occur. Since 2010, reports of pertussis outbreaks have increased, especially in pre-adolescents and teens 10 to 18 years of age. No one knows the exact cause for such outbreaks, but it seems that protection with the acellular vaccine is not as long-lasting as with the older, whole-cell vaccine, and may wane in the pre-adolescent years.

Infants younger than 6 months old are at high risk of severe illness and serious complications. That is because although immunization starts at 2 months of age, the immune response in infants under 6 months is not as strong as in older infants and children, and they may not be fully protected until after their third dose.

Recent recommendations to immunize pregnant women against pertussis may help to prevent infant deaths.

The germ

Bordetella pertussis bacteria were first identified in 1906. Research during the 1970s identified a number of proteins from the cell wall of the bacteria that could both damage the human body and stimulate immune responses. Humans are the only known hosts of these bacteria.

How the germ causes illness

Pertussis is unusual compared with other infections in that the bacteria remain on the surface of a person's airways and do not invade underlying tissue. After exposure, the bacteria attach to cells that line the nose, throat and bronchi (the air tubes in the lungs).

Pertussis toxins damage the cells that line the trachea, making it difficult to clear mucus from the airways. Inflammation causes excess mucus to be made.

The combination of cell damage and excess mucous that stays in the airways causes coughing attacks.

Pertussis toxins also make it difficult for white blood cells to help the body fight infection.

How pertussis spreads

Spread of pertussis requires close contact between people. An infected person may cough or sneeze, spreading droplets with many pertussis bacteria. These droplets can land in the nose or throat of another person who is close by.

A long contagious period. Pertussis is most contagious during the first 2 weeks, when it is often confused with a common cold. It's much less contagious after that, but a person can transmit pertussis for up to 3 weeks after becoming infected. A person is no longer contagious after being treated for 5 days with an appropriate antibiotic.

The illness

Symptoms in children. In most cases, symptoms first occur 9 to 10 days after exposure to the bacteria, but it may take up to 20 days for symptoms to appear. Pertussis usually begins with a runny nose, and there can be quite a bit of discharge. Usually there is no fever, or only a mild one. After a few days to a week, the coughing begins.

Characteristic cough. The cough gets worse and worse until coughing "spells" begin, where the child coughs uncontrollably and cannot take a breath. At the end of a spell, you can hear the characteristic "whoop" sound as the child struggles to take a breath.

Eating, drinking, crying and laughing can all trigger coughing spells. Between spells, a person with pertussis often seems quite normal.

For young infants, these frequent, severe coughing episodes can be exhausting. Babies may even stop breathing due to fatigue. And because they often vomit after coughing and feed poorly when ill, infants can lose weight quickly.

Slow recovery. After 1 to 2 weeks of severe coughing, children begin to get better. Coughing spells gradually go away over the next few weeks. The typical illness lasts 6 to 12 weeks. For several months after recovering from pertussis, children may have coughing spells triggered by anything that irritates their airways, including a common cold, cigarette smoke or breathing cold air.

Pertussis often looks very **different in adolescents and adults**. Almost all have some type of cough, which lasts longer than 3 weeks in most cases (80%) and for 10 weeks or more in half of cases. Although adolescents and adults may not have the "whoop", many will have prolonged coughing spasms which disturb sleep.

Did you know?
The most common source of infection in infants are adolescents and adults living in the same household who have undiagnosed and untreated pertussis.

Complications

Minor complications of pertussis include nosebleeds and small hemorrhages in the white of the eye because of forceful coughing. Pertussis can also cause swelling in the face. Ear infections are very common.

Severe complications. In most children with pertussis, small areas of the lungs collapse because plugs of thick mucus block the airways. These areas are often invaded by other bacteria, which causes pneumonia (infection of the lungs).

About 20% to 30% of infants with pertussis are so sick that they have to stay in hospital. Young infants may have spells when they stop breathing, which can lead to convulsions and coma.

About 1 of every 400 infants hospitalized with pertussis dies, of either pneumonia or brain damage.

About 1 of every 400 infants hospitalized with pertussis suffers brain damage. Pertussis can:
- Interfere with blood supply to the brain during severe coughing spells
- Cause an infant to stop breathing
- Cause the blood vessels in the brain to rupture during coughing spells and bleed into the brain

Studies in Britain show that children who had pertussis in infancy have a much higher rate of learning and behaviour problems later in life than children who never had the infection.

In adolescents and adults. While complications are much less common than in infants, adolescents and adults can be sick for a long time and usually have to take time off from school or work. The intense and persistent coughing can cause sleep disturbances, rib fractures, rectal prolapse and urinary incontinence.

Diagnosis

Bacterial cultures. Most laboratories no longer perform cultures to diagnose pertussis because they are so often negative after a week or two of illness in people who have been vaccinated against pertussis or in people who are only mildly ill.

Also, pertussis bacteria are fragile. The nasal swabs used for culture need specialized handling and transport, and bacteria may not survive in the swab (specimen).

New diagnostic techniques have been developed that are more accurate than performing a culture. These tests find the deoxyribonucleic acid (DNA) of pertussis bacteria in respiratory secretions, and are now routinely used in Canada.

If an adolescent or adult has a cough lasting longer than 2 weeks and there is no other cause identified, it is likely to be pertussis.

Treatment

Antibiotics. Although a number of antibiotics can destroy pertussis bacteria, the results of antibiotic treatment in patients with pertussis have been disappointing. Erythromycin and related antibiotics (though not penicillin, amoxicillin or most other antibiotics) can get rid of pertussis bacteria from the nose and throat but are less likely to have any effect on coughing episodes.

Only early treatment works. If treatment is started in the first 2 weeks of illness, coughing may not last as long. But antibiotics have *no* effect if someone is already experiencing coughing spasms. By this point, the illness is too advanced to respond to treatment. Often, a doctor will try several courses of different antibiotics to stop the cough.

An ounce of prevention...

Preventing pertussis by immunization is safer and more effective than overusing or incorrectly using antibiotics in an attempt to treat this illness.

Post-recovery

A person can get pertussis more than once, but symptoms are usually milder after the first infection. Regardless of how severe the illness is, people with a reinfection are contagious and are a major source of spread, especially to young infants.

Because immunity to pertussis is not lifelong, even people who have had the illness should be fully immunized when they get better.

The vaccine

Type of vaccine

Purified bacterial proteins. The **acellular pertussis vaccine,** used in Canada since 1997–98, is made by extracting and purifying the proteins responsible for inducing immunity.

It is not possible to get pertussis from this vaccine because it contains only purified proteins extracted from the bacteria, and not the bacteria itself.

How pertussis vaccine is made

History of acellular vaccine. The original acellular vaccines, first made in Japan in 1981, consisted of purified extracts of fluid in which pertussis bacteria were grown. Six Japanese manufacturers produced acellular vaccines that varied markedly in composition.

Since then, manufacturers in Canada, the United States and Europe have developed new methods to separate and purify pertussis proteins. Made by various manufacturers, these vaccines differ in both the number and concentration of the proteins in each dose. The vaccines used in Canada contain 3 to 5 purified proteins.

Process. Pertussis bacteria are grown in culture. Their proteins are purified and sterilized, then concentrated. The vaccine is then combined with other vaccines.

For general information on vaccine additives, see Chapter 4.

Available forms of pertussis vaccine

A combined vaccine. In Canada, acellular pertussis vaccine is only available in combination with other vaccines. For more information, see "Vaccines types" in Chapter 4.

Vaccines containing a higher concentration of acellular pertussis antigens are used for infants and for children younger than 7 years of age.

Vaccines containing lower concentrations of pertussis antigens are recommended for older children, adolescents and adults. These lower-dose vaccines are also used for the booster at 4 to 6 years of age in some provinces and territories. Children younger than 4 years old do not respond as well to the lower-dose vaccine.

The antibody response in children 4 years of age and older is similar with the high- and low-dose vaccines. However, because of the reduced amount of pertussis antigens, local reactions such as redness and swelling at the injection site are less frequent with the lower-dose vaccines.

How the vaccine is given

The acellular pertussis-containing vaccines are given by injection into muscle. For more information, see "Getting the shot" in Chapter 4.

Schedule of vaccination

Infants and children (under age 7). For routine immunization of young children in Canada, 4 doses of pertussis vaccine (in combination with other vaccines) are given at 2, 4, 6 and 18 months. A booster dose follows at 4 to 6 years of age. If a dose is missed or delayed for any reason, the missing dose should be given but the series does not have to be started again.

Children (age 7 and over), adolescents and adults. For this group, whether as an initial vaccine or as a booster, a vaccine with a lower dose of acellular pertussis antigens is used.

Boosters (to enhance prior vaccinations)

For adolescents. Teenagers (14 to 16 years of age) in Canada routinely receive a booster dose of acellular pertussis vaccine, which should decrease school outbreaks and disease in this age group and reduce the spread of infection to unimmunized infants.

For adults. It is also recommended that all adults receive at least one booster dose of acellular pertusis vaccine.

During pregnancy. A booster dose in pregnancy provides a high level of antibody against pertussis that will pass from mother to fetus and protect the newborn in the first few months of life. Pregnant women who have not received an adult booster should have pertussis vaccine after their 26th week of pregnancy.

During an outbreak, pertussis vaccine may be given to all pregnant women who may have been exposed to infection, regardless of their immunization history.

> **A booster dose of pertusis vaccine in pregnancy helps to protect the newborn**
>
> Preventing pertussis is especially important in parents and caregivers, who may unknowingly spread the virus to infants.

Length of protection not definitely known. It is not yet clear how long immunity lasts after vaccination with the acellular pertussis vaccine. With the 5-dose schedule used in Canada (at 2, 4, 6 and 18 months and at 4 to 6 years of age), protection should last throughout childhood.

It is expected that the booster doses in adolescence and/or young adulthood will help to extend protection for another 7 to 10 years, but data is still being gathered to determine length of protection.

Possible side effects of pertussis vaccine

Minor side effects of acellular pertussis vaccine usually start within 12 to 24 hours of vaccination. Side effects are much less frequent or severe than those seen with the whole-cell vaccine used before 1997–98.

Generalized side effects in infants may include fever, fussiness, crying, drowsiness, reduced appetite and vomiting. These effects are usually mild and occur in about half of vaccinated infants.

Localized side effects (e.g., redness, swelling, pain and tenderness at the injection site) occur singly or in combination in most infants. These effects are usually mild, last 1 to 2 days, and do not affect behaviour.

With the booster at 4 to 6 years of age, about 1 in 5 children have a larger local reaction, consisting of redness and swelling at the injection site that is larger than 5 cm (2 inches) in size. However, severe pain even with a larger reaction is uncommon: only 1% to 2% of children experience pain that limits arm movement.

A few children develop a firm lump at the injection site, which may not appear for days or weeks. The lump is caused by inflammation and almost always disappears with time.

Both generalized and localized side effects are usually mild.

Severe reactions to pertussis vaccine, such as a high fever (39°C or more), a febrile seizure, prolonged crying and extreme fussiness, are rare.

Hypotensive-hyporesponsive events, where an infant becomes limp, less responsive and pale, have been reported after pertussis vaccines. These reactions are now very rare with today's vaccines but were more common with older pertussis vaccines, which contained whole inactive bacteria. These reactions are probably a response to pain and have no long-term effects.

For more information on possible reactions after receiving a combined vaccine, see Chapter 6, Adverse events and common concerns.

Unfounded concerns

A number of conditions have been blamed on pertussis vaccine. To this day, however, allegations of the dangers of pertussis vaccine are based on anecdote (personal stories) and have not been confirmed by scientific studies.

Studies don't support a causal relationship. Since no form of testing can identify pertussis vaccine as the cause of encephalopathy or any other rare, severe problem, scientists and researchers can only compare how often a particular condition occurs in vaccinated and unvaccinated children. If the rates are the same for both groups of children, it is very unlikely that the vaccine caused the problem.

Brain dysfunction. Acute encephalopathy is a condition where signs of abnormal brain function develop suddenly, including some or all of the following: seizures, aggressiveness, psychosis, stupor or coma. Before the introduction of acellular pertussis vaccine, there were many reports in the medical and mainstream media of acute transient encephalopathy following pertussis vaccine. However, such reports by themselves provide no evidence implicating pertussis vaccine as the cause, and more detailed studies were carried out.

The National Childhood Encephalopathy Study in the United Kingdom found that there might be a slightly increased risk of acute encephalopathy following pertussis vaccine. However, their study could not show whether there was an increased risk of permanent brain damage. Other studies concluded that if brain damage ever occurred after pertussis vaccine, it was an extremely rare event: less than one in one million cases.

On the basis of strong scientific studies, expert groups in Canada (such as the Canadian Paediatric Society and the National Advisory Committee on Immunization), the United States (the American Academy of Pediatrics and Institute of Medicine), the United Kingdom (the British Paediatric Association and British Vaccine Injury Compensation Program) and Australia (the Australian Pediatric Association) all agree that there is no scientific evidence that pertussis vaccine causes brain damage.

Since the combined acellular pertussis vaccine was approved for use in Canada in 1997, no cases of encephalopathy related to this vaccine have been identified by the IMPACT program among children hospitalized with acute neurological illness. (For more information on IMPACT, see Chapter 5, Vaccine Safety and Effectiveness.)

Infantile spasms are another neurological condition in infants that has been blamed on pertussis vaccine. About 150 infants in Canada are affected by this seizure disorder every year. The seizures are complex and difficult to control. Most children with the disorder experience permanent disabilities, including cerebral palsy, delayed development and/or mental retardation.

Infantile spasms usually begin between 2 and 8 months of age, around the same time as infants receive their first 3 doses of pertussis vaccine (at 2, 4 and 6 months). It can therefore be expected that the onset of infantile spasms (an uncommon event) will sometimes coincide with pertussis vaccination (a common event).

Because babies with infantile spasms seem normal in the first few months of life, parents look for an external influence occurring after birth, such as a vaccine, to pinpoint as the cause. However, brain scans reveal that many children with infantile spasms have malformations of the brain that clearly occurred before birth, and it is these malformations that cause the symptoms of this condition.

In Denmark before 1970, the first dose of pertussis vaccine was given at 5 months of age. After 1970, the age at which the first dose should be given was lowered to 5 weeks of age. There was no change in the age of onset of infantile spasms following the change in vaccination schedule. The National Childhood Encephalopathy Study in the United Kingdom. found that children who developed infantile spasms were *less likely* to have received pertussis vaccine within the last 28 days than children who did not develop infantile spasms.

These and other studies were unable to find any evidence to suggest that pertussis vaccine causes infantile spasms.

Sudden infant death syndrome (SIDS). Finally, pertussis vaccine has been blamed for many cases of SIDS. About 2,500 infants die of SIDS every year in the United States. Since most of these deaths occur before 6 months of age, it is to be expected that some of the children had been vaccinated shortly before they died.

The association between vaccination and SIDS is purely coincidental. No large-scale scientific study has confirmed an association between SIDS and vaccination. In fact, scientific studies in the United States, England and France found that infants who died of SIDS were *less likely* to have been vaccinated than infants in the control group (infants in the study who did not die).

In Sweden, no change in the incidence of SIDS was observed following the discontinuation or decrease of pertussis vaccination in 1979. Similarly, in Japan and England, there was no change in the number of SIDS cases when vaccination rates declined in the 1970s.

In the United States and other countries, the number of SIDS deaths has decreased markedly in recent years even though more children are being vaccinated with pertussis vaccine than ever before. The decrease in cases involving SIDS is due to the success of the "Back to Sleep" campaign, which advises parents to place their babies on their backs for sleeping (rather than on their tummies, as was the practice formerly endorsed by paediatricians).

Remember

The Institute of Medicine in the U.S. concluded that there is no causal relationship between pertussis vaccine and death from SIDS or death from any other cause.

Critics of vaccination often claim that pertussis vaccine is the cause of many other conditions, including autism, behavioural disorders, learning disorders, hyperactivity, cancer, leukemia and almost every other illness affecting children. There are no data to support any of these claims.

For more information, see "Vaccine fears" in Chapter 6.

Reasons to delay or avoid pertussis vaccine

For general information on reasons to delay or avoid a vaccine or vaccines, see Chapter 6.

The results of vaccination

Great success with acellular vaccine. Routine use of acellular pertussis vaccine has had great benefits, and the effectiveness of the vaccine has been demonstrated in many ways.

Controlled research trials in Canada comparing the frequency of disease in vaccinated and unvaccinated children have shown that the acellular pertussis vaccine protected 85% of vaccinated children against illness, defined as coughing spells lasting 21 days or more.

The pertussis vaccine does not always prevent infection, especially in people who received vaccine many years before. However, the illness is much milder in previously vaccinated people who become infected.

A marked decline in cases. The routine vaccination of infants and young children has significantly reduced the frequency of pertussis in every country where vaccination programs have been introduced. While it is true that the *number of infant deaths* from pertussis had declined in Canada, the United States and Western Europe long before pertussis vaccine was available, the decline in the *number of cases* only began after mass vaccination was introduced.

Learning from others' experience

The benefits of routine vaccination against pertussis have been confirmed by experience in Japan, Russia, Sweden and the United Kingdom. Significant outbreaks occurred in these countries when their vaccine programs were interrupted.

Outbreaks in other countries. Routine pertussis vaccination began in **Japan** in 1950. Before that, there had been more than 100,000 pertussis cases every year. By 1974, the number had decreased to about 200–400 cases per year. In 1975, the use of pertussis vaccine was halted following the death of two infants who had received a vaccine which contained whole-cell (not acellular) pertussis vaccine.

The ban against pertussis vaccine was lifted 2 months later, when these deaths were determined to have been caused by something other than the vaccine. However, many parents still refused to have their children vaccinated; they were frightened by the publicity surrounding the deaths. The vaccination rate fell from 90% to less than 40%.

In the 4 years before the temporary ban, there were, at most, only 400 cases and 2 to 3 deaths per year from pertussis. After the ban and the ensuing drop in the vaccination rate, an epidemic of pertussis occurred between 1976 and 1979, with over 13,000 cases and more than 100 deaths. Following the introduction of routine immunization with acellular pertussis, the rates of pertussis in Japan returned to levels similar to those seen before 1974.

The use of pertussis vaccine in **Sweden** was discontinued in 1979 because of concern regarding its efficacy and safety. Soon after, the number of cases of pertussis increased markedly: the rate of pertussis in Sweden skyrocketed to 10 times the rate in Canada. Over 60% of children got pertussis before turning 10 years of age. After routine immunization against pertussis started again in the 1990s, using acellular pertussis vaccine, the rate of pertussis declined dramatically.

Before 1970, the rate of pertussis was very low in **England and Wales** because of high rates of immunization. However, following news stories in the early 1970s of the alleged dangers of pertussis vaccine, vaccination rates there declined from 75% to about 25% by 1975.

Two large epidemics of pertussis occurred between 1977 and 1979 and 1981 and 1982. There were more than 100 deaths from pertussis during the first outbreak. When occurrence rates in different parts of the United Kingdom were compared, areas with low rates of vaccination had high rates of pertussis, and vice versa. Once immunization rates increased— following scientific studies of side effects and extensive public education —the rates of pertussis declined to very low levels.

Protection is effective but not long-lasting. Protection from pertussis vaccine may not last forever. In fact, studies of acellular pertussis vaccine suggest that immunity may not last longer than 5 to 7 years after the last dose of vaccine. Such loss of immunity would explain why pertussis is so common in adults.

Studies in Canada, the United States and Australia have shown that 20% to 25% of young adults with a cough lasting more than 2 weeks have pertussis, in spite of having been vaccinated in childhood. Just as with the vaccine, immunity after pertussis infection also declines over time. Although most reinfections with pertussis are mild, full-blown pertussis can occur a second time. Regardless of the severity of the second attack, people who are reinfected with pertussis are very contagious and a major source of spread to others, especially young infants.

The large number of pertussis cases in teens and young adults explains why the disease continues to occur despite the widespread vaccination of infants and young children.

Boosters for adolescents and adults will provide longer lasting protection. Increasing numbers of outbreaks in pre-teens may require, in future, giving the adolescent dose at an earlier age.

Benefits of protection. The major benefit of acellular pertussis vaccine is that it reduces the severity of illness and the risk of complications. Since the risk of complications from the disease is highest in infants younger than 6 months of age, it is important to begin vaccination as early as possible, which is at 2 months of age.

Evidence that pertussis vaccine works:
- Cases of pertussis and related deaths have declined in all countries where the immunization of infants and children is routine.
- Epidemics of pertussis occurred in Japan, Russia, Sweden and the United Kingdom after immunization rates dropped, followed by control of these outbreaks with mass immunization.
- Controlled studies have shown an 85% reduction in the number of pertussis cases in fully immunized children.
- People who are fully immunized have milder disease and fewer complications.

- In Canada, the incidence of pertussis decreased in all age groups between 2005 and 2011, following the introduction of a single adolescent dose of acellular pertussis vaccine.

Snapshots

- Pertussis is a severe disease in young infants. About 1 in 400 infants with pertussis dies, and 1 in 400 suffers permanent brain damage.
- Complications (such as ear infections and pneumonia) are common. Even without complications, infants are sick for 3 to 12 weeks.
- Pertussis vaccine does not always prevent infection. However, it is very effective in reducing the severity of illness and the risk of complications.
- Pertussis is much less common in countries where all infants are routinely immunized.
- All infants and young children should receive pertussis vaccine, and all adolescents should receive a booster dose.
- All adults, especially those in contact with young infants, should receive a booster dose of vaccine to reduce the risk of exposing infants too young to be immunized for pertussis.
- Immunizing pregnant women who have not received an adult booster dose will protect them from pertussis and provide high levels of antibody to their newborns.
- Minor side effects are common with the current vaccine.
- There is no evidence that pertussis vaccine causes brain damage, SIDS, developmental delay, autism, attention-deficit disorder, behavioural disorders, learning disorders, hyperactivity, cancer, leukemia, or any other severe or chronic condition.

18

Pneumococcal disease

Pneumococcus (or *Streptococcus pneumoniae*) is a germ that causes many bacterial infections in children and some in adults. Pneumococcal illnesses, which include ear infections, occur most often in the first two years of life, but they can happen at any age. Pneumococcal illnesses are usually not serious and sometimes go away without antibiotics. Some pneumococcal infections, however, are invasive and very serious. Pneumococcal meningitis (an infection of the brain) can cause brain damage, deafness or even death.

There are more than 90 different types of pneumococci, and a healthy person can get many pneumococcal infections during a lifetime. That's because being immune to one type of pneumococcus does not protect against infections with other types. Certain types cause a lot more disease than others. For example, over 90% of all pneumococcal infections are caused by just 23 types.

Penicillin used to be an effective treatment for all infections caused by pneumococci, but some strains are now resistant to antibiotics, making them more difficult to treat.

> **A germ that causes ear infections can also cause serious illness**
>
> - Pneumococci are the most common cause of meningitis and other serious bacterial infections in children, especially those younger than 2 years old. These germs can also cause serious infections in older children and adults.
> - Pneumococcal infections such as meningitis, septicemia and pneumonia can be fatal. Survivors of meningitis may be left with permanent brain damage or hearing loss.

A history of pneumococcal disease

Before vaccine

Before the conjugate pneumococcal vaccine was introduced in 2001, about 500,000 cases of pneumococcal disease occurred every year in Canada. Many were children under 2 years old, including about:
- 65 with meningitis (infection of the membranes and fluid that cover the brain and spinal cord),
- 700 with bacteremia (infection of the bloodstream),
- 2,200 with pneumonia (infection of the lungs), and
- 200,000 with an ear infection.

After vaccine

The first vaccine against pneumococcus was developed in the late 1940s. It was never widely used because the introduction of penicillin right after World War II made the vaccine seem unnecessary. This vaccine was made from polysaccharides (complex sugars) from only four of the germ types that cause pneumococcal infections.

The current purified polysaccharide vaccine, approved for use in Canada in 1983, contains complex sugars from all 23 types that cause over 90% of serious infections. This vaccine is used mostly in people aged 65 and over and in younger adults and children with medical conditions that put them at risk for serious pneumococcal infection.

The polysaccharide vaccine has been never used routinely in healthy children because it is not believed to be very effective. In fact, it is not effective at all in children under 2 years old.

Fortunately, as with Hib vaccine (see Chapter 9), the new conjugate form of pneumococcal vaccine is very effective in protecting children of all ages. Within three years of the pneumococcal conjugate vaccine being licensed in the United States in 2000, the rate of serious infections caused by the 7 types of pneumococcus in the conjugate vaccine had decreased by 94%.

Immunizing young children in the United States also had a very important indirect effect. Because vaccination reduces the spread of the vaccine-specific pneumococcus types in the whole population, older children, adults and especially the elderly are also protected by lower exposure to the 7 vaccine types. Consequently, the number of cases of invasive pneumococcal disease in the elderly had also decreased 65% by 2003 in the United States.

The conjugate vaccine was approved for use in Canada in 2001, and by 2006 all infants could receive it as part of the routine schedule.

An important impact in Canada!

A study in the Calgary Health Region showed that by 2007, there had been a 79% decline in serious pneumococcal infections in children under 2 years old, as compared with the years before vaccine.

Looking only at serious infections caused by the 7 types in the conjugate vaccine, there was a 94% decline in children under 2 years and a 92% decline in adults 65 to 84 years old.

While the conjugate vaccine was every effective in controlling infections caused by the 7 types it contained, the number of infections due to other types began to increase over the next few years. One of these, 19A, is now the type found most frequently in young children in Canada. In 2010, a newer version of the conjugate vaccine that covers 13 (rather than just 7) types of pneumococcus, including 19A, became available and is now being used across Canada.

The germ

Pneumococcal bacteria infect only humans and cause a wide range of infections. The infection always starts in the nose or throat, where the bacteria attach to cells on the surface of the respiratory tract.

What is "healthy carriage"?

Most people have no symptoms after becoming infected with pneumococci. They become "**carriers**" of a "silent" infection as they host the bacteria in their nose or throat. Pneumococcal carriage can begin early, often in infancy, and continue on and off throughout life. At any given time, up to 40% of all people are healthy carriers of pneumococci.

Pneumococci can infect the lining of a person's nose and throat for weeks or months. This carrier infection triggers an immune response to the specific type being carried, but not to other pneumococcal types. Usually, a person carries one type at a time for several months before developing immunity to it. Soon after, carriage of a new type—and the process of building immunity to it—begin again.

It is not known why one person becomes a silent carrier or gets a mild infection, such as an ear infection, while someone else gets meningitis or another invasive illness after picking up a new pneumococcal type. It is known that people with certain medical conditions are more likely to have serious infections.

How the germ causes illness

Infection and illness. Pneumococcal bacteria have an external coat, or capsule, made of large complex sugars (polysaccharides). This capsule protects the bacteria against attack by white blood cells, our body's main defense against infection. If a person doesn't have antibodies to the type of pneumococcus in their nose and throat, white blood cells can't attack and kill the bacteria. Pneumococci then invade the body, multiply freely and cause disease.

Inside the capsule is the cell wall of the pneumococcus. When substances from this cell wall are released into the body, they cause an intense reaction, called **inflammation**.

How pneumococci spread

Most infections are spread by healthy carriers, but people who are ill can also infect others.

Spread from an infected person to another person requires close contact: through uncovered coughs and sneezes when other people are close by, or a transfer of saliva (e.g., by kissing or mouth-to-mouth sharing of toys, food, cutlery, or items such as a water bottle, drinking straw, toothbrush, cigarette, lipstick, mouthguard, or a musical instrument with a mouthpiece).

Children who attend a child care centre have significantly higher carrier rates of pneumococci than children who are at home. Children are more likely to share mouthed items in a child care setting and are in very close contact with other children during play.

The illness

Two kinds of pneumococcal infection cause symptoms:
• Surface infections of the respiratory tract, which affect the lining of the respiratory tract and the surrounding tissues;

- Invasive infections, which enter the bloodstream and spread to organs and tissues.

Surface infections. When a new type of pneumococci (one against which a person has no immunity) infects the nose and throat, bacteria can cause disease elsewhere in the respiratory tract, often in the ears, sinuses or lungs. About 15% of young children get an **ear infection (acute otitis media)** within one month of being infected with a new type. Ear infections often follow a viral infection of the respiratory tract, such as the common cold. The cold virus can damage cells lining the middle ear, making it easier for pneumococci to get in and cause more damage.

Very few children escape having at least one ear infection in their first 5 years of life. About 20% of children have frequent (recurrent) ear infections, that is, three or more attacks per year. Pneumococci cause 40% to 60% of all ear infections and are the most frequent cause of recurrent ear infections.

Pneumococci are also the most common cause of **acute sinusitis**. Sinusitis is an infection of the sinuses (air-filled spaces inside the bones of the face), and most cases follow a cold. The sinuses connect to the nasal passage by very narrow openings, which can become blocked during a cold, allowing bacteria in the nose to spread into the sinuses. Inflammation and a build-up of pus in the sinuses cause pain, local tenderness and sometimes, fever.

The most serious surface infection of the respiratory tract is **pneumonia**, which involves the alveoli (air spaces in the lungs where oxygen enters the body and carbon dioxide exits). Symptoms are fever, rapid breathing, difficult breathing, a cough that often produces yellow or greenish sputum, and chest pain.

A chest X-ray will show inflammation and an accumulation of fluid and cells in the air spaces of the lung. A few children with pneumococcal pneumonia (less than 1 in 10 cases) have bacteremia (see just below) at the same time as pneumonia.

Invasive infections. When pneumococci spread from the nose and throat into the blood, it is called **bacteremia**. Pneumococcal bacteremia might or might not spread the infection to other organs. In its early stages, bacteremia looks very much like a viral infection, because a high fever is usually the only sign of illness. (More than 95% of children younger than age 2 with high fever have a viral infection, not a serious bacterial infection.) High fever by itself is not harmful.

Septicemia is a much more severe form of bacteremia. Pneumococci grow rapidly in the blood and overwhelm the body. The bacteria also release toxic substances from their cell walls. In high concentrations, they can damage small blood vessels in the skin, heart, lungs, kidneys and other organs. Septicemia can cause shock (a sudden drop in blood pressure), organ failure, and death. Illness is sudden and severe: the total time from the first symptom of fever to death can be as short as 6 to 12 hours.

Pneumococcal septicemia is rare in otherwise healthy people. However, children and adults who do not have a spleen, due to surgery or a birth defect, or whose spleen cannot function normally (e.g., because of sickle-cell anemia) are at much higher risk. The spleen is a filter, helping to remove bacteria from the blood. Without a spleen, bacteria can grow very rapidly to high concentrations. A person who has a spleen but whose immune system is not working well is also at high risk of severe pneumococcal infections.

Infection of other body parts. When pneumococci enter the bloodstream, they can infect almost any other part of the body, often the lungs, central nervous system, joints, bones or peritoneum (lining of the abdominal wall).

Meningitis is caused by bacteria in the blood spreading into the spinal fluid and membranes covering the brain and spinal cord. Blood supply to the brain can be affected by inflammation and blocked blood vessels. Brain cells cannot survive interruption of their blood supply for very long, and inflammation can cause permanent brain damage. Early signs of meningitis can be very similar to those of influenza and other viral infections. This makes diagnosis difficult, especially in infants. The symptoms of meningitis are summarized in Table 18.1.

Table 18.1
Symptoms of pneumococcal meningitis

In older children and adults	In babies
High fever	Fever
Drowsiness or impaired consciousness	Difficult to wake up
Irritability, fussiness, agitation	Fretfulness or irritability, especially when handled
Severe headache	Difficulty feeding
Vomiting	Vomiting
Stiff neck	Stiff neck and bulging of the fontanelle (the soft spot on top of the head) may occur in young babies, but usually very late in the illness
Pain when moving neck	Not usually present

Complications

Surface infections. If children get their first ear infection before they turn a year old, there's a high probability they'll have several more over the next few years. An ear infection can be complicated by a perforated eardrum, which, if it does not heal on its own, may require surgery. Rarely, the infection spreads from the ear to the bone behind the ear, causing **acute mastoiditis**, which sometimes requires surgery. Also, rarely, ear infections can spread to the brain.

Invasive infections. These can be very severe. About 10% of patients with pneumococcal **meningitis** die, even with appropriate treatment. Deafness occurs in 5% to 10% of survivors of meningitis, and permanent brain damage occurs in another 10% to 15%. Pneumococcal **septicemia** can be fatal in all age groups. Pneumococcal **pneumonia** is a common cause of death in the elderly.

Diagnosis

Tests are needed. Diagnosing pneumococcal disease depends on finding the bacteria in the blood, cerebrospinal fluid or infected tissues. Meningitis can only be confirmed by performing a lumbar puncture—inserting a small needle into the spinal canal in the lower back and removing a sample of fluid. This fluid is examined in the laboratory for bacteria and for signs of inflammation, such as more white blood cells than normal and changes in concentrations of protein and sugar.

Treatment

Antibiotics. A leading reason that doctors prescribe antibiotics for children is to treat suspected or proven pneumococcal infections, especially otitis media. *Healthy carriers of pneumococcus do not need antibiotics.* Surface infections with pneumococcus, such as sinusitis or an ear infection, may get better on their own, though many cases require antibiotics. Antibiotics are usually given by mouth. Some children with pneumonia are too sick to be treated by mouth and require intravenous treatment (through a needle in a vein).

All invasive infections require antibiotics, usually given intravenously.

Before antibiotics, pneumococcal meningitis was always fatal. With antibiotic treatment, the death rate has been reduced to about 10%. A delay in diagnosing and treating meningitis increases the risk of deafness and brain damage.

Post-recovery

Immunity after infection is only for the pneumococcal type that caused the infection. Therefore, being vaccinated is an essential step toward developing immunity against other types.

The vaccine

Types of vaccines

There are two types of pneumococcal vaccines, both made from purified complex sugars extracted from the bacteria. Because the vaccines are highly purified extracts and do not contain whole bacteria, it is impossible to get the disease or symptoms of the disease from the vaccine.

Pneumococcal polysaccharide vaccine (PPV23) contains 23 types of pneumococci. Polysaccharides protect bacteria from being attacked and destroyed by white blood cells. As vaccines, they help trigger the human immune response. Antibodies combine with polysaccharides to coat the surface of bacteria, making it easy for the white blood cells to ingest and kill them.

Children under 2 years old do not respond to vaccines containing polysaccharide alone.

The first **pneumococcal conjugate vaccine (PVC7)**, with 7 types of pneumococci, was approved for use in Canada in 2001. A vaccine covering 10 types (PVC10) was approved in 2009 and the one now in use, covering 13 types, was approved in 2010. Like the Hib and meningococcal conjugate vaccines (see Chapters 9 and 15), the pneumococcal conjugates are made from purified polysaccharides, which are chemically linked to a purified protein. (Conjugate means "joined together".)

Linking the purified sugar to a protein carrier creates a vaccine that is much more effective in young children, including infants.

The 13 pneumococcal types in PCV13, the vaccine now used in Canada, were chosen from the more than 90 possible serotypes of pneumococci because they cause most invasive pneumococcal infections in infants and young children in Canada and the United States.

How pneumococcal vaccines are made

Process for pneumococcal polysaccharide vaccine. The vaccine for each of the 23 types of pneumococci is prepared separately. Pneumococcal bacteria are grown in liquid culture. When growth is complete, the bacteria are removed and the polysaccharide is extracted and purified. The 23 different sugars used in the purified polysaccharide vaccine are combined in the final product.

Process for pneumococcal conjugate vaccine. To make the conjugate vaccine, the purified polysaccharides of the 13 chosen types of pneumococci are prepared, then chemically linked to a protein. The protein, called CRM, is highly purified and very similar to diphtheria toxoid.

For general information on vaccine additives, see Chapter 4.

Available forms of pneumococcal vaccine

Not combined. Neither the polysaccharide vaccine nor the conjugate vaccine is available in combination with other vaccines.

Vaccines for different age groups. The conjugate vaccine is the only type of pneumococcal vaccine that is effective in children under 2 years old.

The polysaccharide vaccine is only given to children with specific medical problems who are at least 2 years old and have already received all recommended doses of the conjugate vaccine.

Although the polysaccharide vaccine covers 23 types and the conjugate vaccine covers only 13 types, children have a better immune response to the conjugate vaccine. Therefore, it makes sense to give both vaccines to children with a chronic medical problem that makes them vulnerable to pneumococcal infections (see the text box in "Schedule of vaccination", below).

PPV23 is also given to adolescents and adults with specific medical problems and to all adults aged 65 years and over.

How the vaccines are given

Both the polysaccharide and conjugate vaccines are given by injection into muscle. The polysaccharide vaccine can also be given subcutaneously (beneath the skin). For more information, see "Getting the shot" in Chapter 4.

Schedule of vaccination

Conjugate vaccine

Children under age 2. The National Advisory Committee on Immunization recommends routine immunization of all children younger than

2 years of age with the pneumococcal conjugate vaccine. The schedule is summarized in Table 18.2.

Children 2 to 5 years old. Vaccination with the conjugate vaccine is recommended for all children 24 to 59 months (5 years) of age who were not vaccinated as infants. There is a moderate risk of invasive pneumococcal disease in this age group. Children in any child care setting are at higher risk of pneumococcal disease than children who stay at home, but *all* children 2 to 5 years of age are at some risk and therefore benefit from receiving the vaccine.

Table 18.2
Recommended schedule for pneumococcal conjugate vaccine in children under 5 years old

Age at first dose	Primary series**	Booster dose
2 to 11 months, otherwise healthy	2 doses, *at least* 8 weeks apart	1 dose at 12 to 15 months of age, and at least 8 weeks after the last dose in the primary series
2 to 11 months at increased risk of pneumococcal disease*	3 doses, *at least* 8 weeks apart	
12 to 23 months	2 doses, 8 weeks apart	none
24 to 59 months	1 dose	none

* See text box, below
** The first 2 or 3 doses

Children 5 years of age and older. Children and adolescents at risk of invasive pneumoncoccal disease (see text box, below) who have not previously received the conjugate vaccine should receive one dose.

Healthy children and adolescents in this age group do not need pneumococcal vaccine.

Adults. A single dose of conjugate vaccine is recommended for adults with immune system disorders (see text box, below).

Polysaccharide vaccine

Pneumococcal polysaccharide vaccine is recommended for people at risk of severe or fatal pneumococcal infections, namely:

- Children over 2 years old, adolescents and adults who have any of the chronic medical problems listed in the text box, below.
- All adults age 65 years and older.

Both vaccines

Children at high risk for serious pneumococcal disease need both vaccines

The conjugate vaccine stimulates immune memory and gives a better antibody response to the 13 types that are in it, but the polysaccharide vaccine also works against another 10 types that are not in the conjugate vaccine.

If both conjugate and polysaccharide vaccines are needed, the polysaccharide vaccine should be given *at least* 8 weeks after the last dose of conjugate vaccine. For more information, see Chapter 3, When extra protection is needed.

Boosters (to enhance prior vaccinations). Booster doses of the **conjugate vaccine** are not needed once the appropriate number of doses for age and condition have been given.

A booster dose of **polysaccharide vaccine**, 5 years after the first, is recommended for people at high risk of invasive pneumococcal disease. An earlier booster may be needed for bone marrow or stem cell transplant recipients. People over 65 years of age who are otherwise healthy do not need a booster.

Length of protection. How long a person is protected after receiving the **polysaccharide vaccine** is not known. The **conjugate vaccine** produces a high level of protection against disease caused by the 13 serotypes in the vaccine. Because the conjugate vaccine induces immune memory, protection is expected to last many years, if not for life.

Medical conditions that increase the risk of invasive pneumococcal disease

- Disorders of the immune system:
  - Sickle cell disease and certain other congenital disorders of hemoglobin (red blood cells)
  - Absent spleen or a spleen that does not work well because of congenital defect, disease or surgery
  - Conditions or treatments that weaken the immune system, including congenital conditions, cancer, HIV infection, or transplantation of bone marrow, stem cells or an organ
- Other conditions:
  - Chronic heart or lung disease, including asthma requiring medical care in the preceding 12 months
  - Chronic neurologic conditions that impair clearance of oral secretions
  - Diabetes (type 1 and 2)
  - Chronic kidney disease, including nephrotic syndrome
  - Chronic liver disease
  - Chronic cerebrospinal fluid leak
  - Cochlear implants, including children who are to receive implants

---

Possible side effects of pneumococcal vaccines

The pneumococcal polysaccharide vaccine is very safe. Between 30% to 60% of people who get this shot experience redness, swelling, pain and tenderness at the injection site. Local reactions happen more often when the vaccine is injected under the skin rather than into muscle but are rarely severe. Fever and other general reactions are uncommon. The vaccine has not been shown to cause any serious adverse events. It can be given at the same time as other childhood vaccines.

The pneumococcal conjugate vaccine is also very safe. About 20% to 30% of people who get this shot have mild local reactions (e.g., redness, swelling, soreness) and a low-grade fever for a day or two. Local reactions after this vaccine, especially redness, happen more often than after routine infant/childhood combination vaccines. However, more general reactions, such as fever and irritability are *not* more frequent or severe when the pneumococcal conjugate vaccine is given at the same time as a combination vaccine.

Reasons to delay or avoid pneumococcal vaccine

For general information on reasons to delay or avoid a vaccine or vaccines, see Chapter 6.

The results of vaccination

- All studies to date have shown a dramatic drop in the number of invasive infections caused by the pneumococcus types found in the conjugate vaccine.
- Studies have noted a higher number of infections caused by pneumococcus types *not* found in the conjugate vaccine against 7 types, but it seems hopeful that the conjugate vaccine with 13 types will overcome this problem.
- The conjugate vaccine decreases the number of ear infections and pneumonia cases in young children. It probably also prevents some sinus infections, but this has not been studied.
- The conjugate vaccine also decreases healthy carriage of the pneumococcus types contained in the vaccine. This helps to explain the declining number of cases of invasive pneumococcal disease in the elderly, who might otherwise get an infection from their grandchildren.
- There is less data on the effectiveness of polysaccharide vaccine. Some studies show a lower number of invasive pneumococcal infections in people with HIV infection and in the elderly, but protection varies. More studies of the effectiveness of polysaccharide vaccine in children with chronic medical problems are needed.

Snapshots

- Both the purified pneumococcal polysaccharide vaccine and the pneumococcal conjugate vaccine are very safe.

- Pneumococcal vaccines have dramatically reduced both local and invasive forms of infection in all age groups.
- Routinely immunizing children younger than 2 years old with the pneumococcal conjugate vaccine has been very effective for:
  - preventing bacteremia and meningitis caused by pneumococcal types contained in the vaccine;
  - reducing rates of ear infections and pneumonia caused by vaccine types;
  - decreasing the use of antibiotics by preventing ear infections and pneumonia, and possibly sinus infections;
  - reducing healthy carriage of vaccine types, and thereby reducing spread of these types to older children and adults;
  - preventing invasive meningitis and bacteremia in older people, an indirect effect of reduced spread of vaccine serotypes.
- Routinely immunizing people of all ages who are at higher risk of invasive pneumococcal disease has also reduced rates of death and severe disease in this population.

19

Polio

Polio (short for poliomyelitis) is an infection caused by poliovirus. Most infections with poliovirus occur without illness. In its most severe form, however, poliovirus can infect and destroy nerve cells in the spinal cord that control muscle contraction. When these nerve cells die, muscles become weak or paralyzed. The nerve damage is permanent.

A history of polio

Before vaccine

A global disease. Paralytic polio used to be the most common infectious cause of major crippling disease in the world.

Polio cases occurred year-round in the tropics and during the summer and fall in more temperate regions of the world. Until about 100 years ago, almost all infants became infected with polio. But even then, infection resulted in paralytic polio only infrequently. That's because young infants were partly protected by antibodies passed on to them by their mothers.

As sanitation conditions and hygiene improved during the late 19th and early 20th centuries, the risk of exposure to poliovirus shifted from early childhood (infants and young children) to later childhood. Older children, adolescents and adults were more likely to suffer paralysis from the infection than younger children. Most children were not immune, so the virus flourished whenever it was introduced into a community. During this time in North America and Western Europe, epidemics of paralytic polio began to occur, especially in urban areas.

The last major epidemics in North America were between 1951 and 1954, just before polio vaccine became available. There were over 65,000 cases of paralytic polio in the United States alone. The last major epidemic in Canada was in 1959, with nearly 2,000 cases. In that outbreak, the rate of paralytic disease was highest in children 5 to 9 years old. However, paralytic polio also occurred in adolescents and adults: over one-third of cases in Canada and the United States were in people over the age of 15.

After vaccine

A significant drop in cases. In 1955, more than 76,000 cases of paralytic polio were reported in Canada, the United States, the former Soviet Union, Western Europe, Australia and New Zealand. That year, inactivated polio vaccine (IPV) was used for the first time. In 1967, there were only 1,013 cases in these same countries—a reduction of almost 99% in just 12 years!

Polio can cause severe illness
- One in every 100 people who get polio develop paralysis.
- Some people who have paralytic polio develop post-polio syndrome many years later.

The incidence of paralytic polio has continued to fall in all countries with successful vaccination programs. The last case of paralytic polio due to wild (naturally occurring) poliovirus in Canada was in 1989.

The global campaign to eradicate polio, promoted by UNICEF and the World Health Organization (WHO), has been remarkably successful. The WHO estimates there were 350,000 cases of paralytic polio in 1988. But between 2011 and 2013, reported cases worldwide averaged just 426 annually, a reduction of 99.8%!

Poliovirus has been eradicated from the entire Western Hemisphere: the last known case of disease due to wild poliovirus occurred in Peru in 1991. Poliovirus has also been eradicated from most other countries.

In 2014, wild poliovirus continues to spread and cause disease in only three countries: Afghanistan, Nigeria and Pakistan. But poliovirus from these countries continues to spread into neighbouring countries. For example, an outbreak of paralytic disease due to wild poliovirus occurred in Nigeria in 2005, after religious leaders led a campaign against the vaccination program. It spread to many countries in Africa and Indonesia and affected over 1,000 children. Outbreaks occurred in Europe in 2010 after the disruption of certain health care programs caused immunization rates to fall. Outbreaks continue to occur in areas of conflict and population displacement.

Mass vaccination programs in developing countries could make global eradication a reality. Major efforts are underway to ensure eradication by 2018. Until the virus has been eliminated worldwide, children in Canada must continue to be immunized. The risk of travellers bringing polioviruses back into Canada is too great to ignore.

Polio can be erradicated

Because poliovirus, like smallpox, infects only humans, the disease can be eradicated if all children are vaccinated. Once all people are immune, the vaccine will no longer be needed.

But as long as a single child remains infected, children in all countries are at risk of contracting polio.

The germ

The poliovirus was first identified in the laboratory in 1949. There are three different types of poliovirus, based on proteins located in the external coat of the virus.

How the germ causes illness

After entering the body, poliovirus infects cells in the throat and intestinal tract. The virus multiplies and spreads through the blood to the spinal cord and brain. Within the spinal cord, the virus moves along nerve fibres. If a large amount of virus grows in the spinal cord, nerve cells that activate muscles are destroyed. Depending on the extent of nerve cell damage, weakness or complete paralysis of muscles can occur.

How polio spreads

Poliovirus is found in the throat and feces of infected people. It usually spreads to others when hands, water or food become contaminated with feces. Less often, it is spread directly from the throat.

Fecal contamination. The virus in feces can spread because of poor hygiene and inadequate sanitation. An infected person who does not wash hands thoroughly after going to the bathroom can spread the virus by touching others or by contact with food, water and objects. Inadequate sewage treatment can lead to environmental contamination, especially of a water supply. When a water supply becomes contaminated, the virus can spread to many people.

From the throat. Spread of poliovirus requires close contact between people. An infected person's cough or sneeze can spread droplets containing many virus particles to the nose or throat of another person.

All individuals infected with polio are contagious, regardless of how severe their illness is. Virus is shed (or released) from the throat for 1 to 2 weeks, and in the stool for 4 to 8 weeks, after infection.

People with mild or no illness can still spread the virus to others

The spread of polio was a mystery until it was discovered that only 1 in every 100 infected people develops paralytic disease. Transmission by people who were not known to have polio explained the rapid spread of infection.

The illness

Symptoms. The time between infection and the start of symptoms is usually 7 to 14 days. About 90% to 95% of infected people have no symptoms at all. In another 4% to 8%, the only sign of infection is a minor illness lasting a few days, with one or more of the following symptoms: fever, sore throat, muscle aches and pains, drowsiness, headache, loss of appetite, nausea, vomiting, abdominal pain and constipation.

In 1% to 5% of cases, symptoms indicating spread of virus to the spinal cord and/or brain develop 1 to 2 days later. This form of the infection is called viral or aseptic meningitis. The person experiences neck stiffness, severe headache, vomiting and lethargy or drowsiness because the membranes and fluid covering the brain and spinal cord become inflamed. This illness lasts 2 to 10 days, and is followed by rapid and complete recovery.

Severe illness. Only about 1 out of every 100 people infected with the virus gets **paralytic polio**, the most severe form of disease. Sudden muscle weakness or paralysis occurs in various body parts, progressing rapidly over a few days. Often there is severe pain in non-paralyzed muscles. While some recovery of muscle function may occur after infection, most people with this form of disease are permanently paralyzed.

Paralysis usually affects one part of the body more than others, and leg paralysis is much more common than arm paralysis. In a few cases, the diaphragm and chest muscles are paralyzed, making it difficult or impossible to breathe. These individuals need a mechanical ventilator to survive.

Complications

Death from paralytic polio can result from damage to the nerve centres that control breathing, blood circulation and other vital functions. People who need a mechanical ventilator to breathe are at higher risk for developing pneumonia, which can cause death.

Post-polio syndrome. Some people who have had paralytic polio experience a progression of muscle pain, weakness and paralysis later in life—a condition called post-polio syndrome. The interval between the original illness and the onset of new symptoms can be as long as 15 to 40 years.

An estimated one-quarter of paralytic polio cases may develop post-polio syndrome. It is not possible for the poliovirus itself to cause new disease because it is no longer present. Post-polio syndrome is probably caused by the overuse or aging of damaged muscles.

Diagnosis

Tests are needed. The diagnosis of polio depends on finding the virus in throat, feces or cerebrospinal fluid samples. Blood tests to detect an increase in specific antibody to poliovirus can aid diagnosis but are less useful.

Treatment

Supportive treatments. There is no cure for polio or the paralysis it produces, but supportive treatments such as warm baths, massage and physiotherapy can help to relieve muscle pain during the acute illness and prevent complications. Long-term care and rehabilitation can help individuals live with paralysis.

Post-recovery

Immunity develops after infection, but only to the type of poliovirus that caused the infection. Repeat attacks of paralytic polio are extremely rare.

The vaccine

Types of vaccines

There are two different kinds of polio vaccine: inactivated polio vaccine (IPV), which contains killed, intact virus; and oral polio vaccine (OPV), which contains live, attenuated (weakened) virus. Both vaccines contain the three polioviruses, types 1, 2 and 3. Today, only IPV is used in Canada and the United States.

IPV contains only killed virus and cannot cause paralytic polio.

OPV contains live strains of poliovirus that have been weakened in the laboratory.

OPV was used before 1997–98 in British Columbia, Alberta, Saskatchewan, Manitoba, Quebec and New Brunswick. Because the weakened vaccine strains have not *completely* lost the ability to damage nerve cells, there is a very small risk of getting paralytic polio after receiving OPV. OPV is no longer used in Canada because the few cases of paralytic polio from 1980 to 1995 were associated with this vaccine.

OPV vaccine continues to be widely used internationally. This vaccine is less expensive to make and easier to use because it is given by mouth. OPV is also more effective than IPV in controlling virus transmission: it prevents the polio virus from growing in the intestine and, as a result, being excreted into the environment.

How polio vaccines are made

Process for making IPV. Poliovirus is produced using either a human cell line (MRC-5 cells) or a cell line derived from monkey kidneys (Vero cells). The MRC-5 cells are descended from cells taken decades ago from a single human fetus. The Vero cells come from monkeys born and raised in special breeding facilities. These cell lines are grown under controlled conditions and stored in freezers until they are needed. All of the cells used to make polio vaccines today have been studied for many years. They are tested repeatedly to make sure no contaminating viruses are present.

Poliovirus particles are separated from the cells, purified and concentrated, then treated with formaldehyde to inactivate (kill) the virus. The final product contains all three types of poliovirus.

For general information on vaccine additives, see Chapter 4.

Available forms of polio vaccine

IPV is available in Canada both as a single vaccine and in combination with two or more other vaccines.

OPV is no longer available in Canada.

How the vaccine is given

IPV is given by injection into muscle. For more information, see "Getting the shot" in Chapter 4.

Schedule of vaccination

Infants and children (under age 7). For routine immunization of young children in Canada, 4 doses of IPV (in combination with other vaccines) are given at 2, 4, 6 and 18 months of age, with a booster at 4 to 6 years of age. If a dose is missed or delayed for any reason, the missing dose should be given but the series does not have to be started again.

Children (age 7 and over) and adolescents. The schedule for older children and adolescents not previously immunized is 2 doses of a vaccine containing IPV, given 4 to 8 weeks apart, followed by a booster 6 to 12 months later.

Adults (18 years of age and older). Unimmunized adults who are at higher risk of polio exposure should get 2 doses of a vaccine containing IPV, given 4 to 8 weeks apart, followed by a booster 6 to 12 months later. Those at higher risk include:
- Travellers to areas where polio is present,
- People in close contact with others who may be excreting poliovirus or OPV, notably
  - people working with refugees,

- health care workers,
- contacts of internationally adopted infants and other children who may have received OPV
- Laboratory workers.

Unimmunized adults who are not at higher risk may be given IPV in combination with their next tetanus and diphtheria booster.

Boosters (to enhance prior vaccinations). Additional doses of IPV are not needed by adolescents or adults who have been fully immunized unless they are at higher risk of exposure (as above), in which case a single lifetime booster dose of IPV is recommended.

Length of protection. Protection is long-lasting.

Possible side effects of polio vaccines

IPV. This vaccine is very safe. Other than minor pain and redness at the injection site, side effects after IPV are extremely rare.

OPV. Weakening the strains of poliovirus used in OPV greatly reduces their ability to cause nerve damage. Safety tests have shown that compared with wild virus strains, OPV lowers the risk of damage in monkey spinal cords by a factor of at least 1 million. Nevertheless, the potential to cause nerve damage, though extremely remote, is still present.

The risk of vaccine-associated paralytic polio is estimated to be 1 case in 2.7 million doses. The risk for individuals in close contact with an infant vaccinated with OPV is 1 case in over 20 million doses of vaccine.

The decision to stop using OPV in Canada, the United States and several other countries was made for the following reasons:
- IPV prevents paralytic disease caused by wild poliovirus without the risk, however small, of causing paralytic disease.
- The eradication of wild poliovirus from the Western Hemisphere and falling rates elsewhere meant that the risk of exposure to wild poliovirus in Canada was extremely low. Therefore, the risk of paralytic polio from OPV, however small, was higher than the risk of paralysis from wild polio.

Reasons to delay or avoid polio vaccine

For general information on reasons to delay or avoid a vaccine or vaccines, see Chapter 6.

The results of vaccination

IPV

Effective and long-lasting. After 3 doses of IPV, 100% of infants develop protective levels of antibodies against all three types of poliovirus. The boosters given at 18 months and between 4 and 6 years of age ensure that protection lasts for many years.

High levels of protection. Field trials of the original IPV (Salk vaccine) produced between 1955 and 1959 showed that it protected against paralytic polio in 55% of recipients after 1 dose, 80% after 2 doses, 91% after 3 doses, and 96% after 4 doses. Current vaccines are much stronger than the original Salk vaccine and have been shown to be 90% effective after just 2 doses; 100% protection is achieved after the 5 doses recommended in Canada.

Preventing outbreaks. The Canadian experience has demonstrated that paralytic polio can be eliminated with the use of IPV alone.

Over the past 50 years, travellers infected with polio have brought the virus back home. However, only three small outbreaks of paralytic polio have occurred in all that time. The groups of people who became infected had all refused immunization for religious reasons. And while many people came into close contact with these infected individuals, no disease occurred in those who had been vaccinated.

OPV

Effective in eradicating polio. OPV is just as effective as IPV in preventing paralytic disease. OPV is more effective than IPV in controlling virus spread because it prevents polioviruses from growing in the intestine and thus being excreted into the environment.

Mass vaccination programs in developing countries. Because OPV is less expensive and easier to give than IPV, it has been used extensively in developing countries. The approach to eradication of poliovirus has been to vaccinate all children under 5 years of age in these countries with OPV on the same day. A second dose of OPV is given 4 to 6 weeks later, again on the same day.

These mass vaccination programs, promoted by UNICEF and the World Health Organization, are called **National Immunization Days**. Most funding to buy the OPV vaccine for these programs has been provided by Rotary International, but many countries contribute monetarily. The donations of large quantities of OPV by vaccine manufacturers have also been crucial for success. National Immunization Days are a key strategy for eradicating polio worldwide.

Evidence that polio vaccines work:
- Large-scale, controlled field trials of both IPV and OPV have demonstrated that both vaccines prevent infection with wild poliovirus, thereby preventing paralytic disease.
- The number of cases of paralytic polio has decreased by 99.8% worldwide as a result of vaccination.
- Wild poliovirus has been eradicated from all but three countries in the world. Even in those places (Afghanistan, Nigeria and Pakistan), the number of paralytic polio cases has dropped dramatically.
- In several countries, the only cases of paralytic polio over the past 50 years have been in members of small groups of unvaccinated individuals.

Snapshots

- Both IPV and OPV are very effective in preventing paralytic polio and eliminating the spread of wild poliovirus.
- IPV is safer than OPV because it contains no live virus.
- OPV is widely used for massive immunization campaigns in developing countries because it is less expensive and easier to give

than IPV, as well as more effective than IPV for preventing the spread of wild poliovirus.
- Paralytic polio has been eradicated from the most of the world, and with the implementation of National Immunization Days, prospects are very good for global eradication by 2018.
- Until worldwide eradication of polio has been achieved, routine polio vaccination for all children must continue.

20

Rotavirus

Rotavirus is the most common cause of acute diarrhea in infants and young children in the world. The illness causes a great deal of watery diarrhea and vomiting that can quickly lead to dehydration. In Canada, rotavirus causes 10% to 40% of all childhood gastroenteritis (which is sometimes called "stomach flu").

Rotavirus gastroenteritis usually gets better on its own, but it is a costly illness. About one-third of infected children see a doctor; one in 7 goes to an emergency department, and one in 14 is hospitalized. Most children who are hospitalized for gastroenteritis have rotavirus.

In Canada, most cases of rotavirus diarrhea occur in the late winter and early spring. Outbreaks can occur any time between December and May, but infections are uncommon the rest of the year.

In developing countries, more than 400,000 children under the age of 5 die each year from rotavirus diarrhea. This virus **kills one in 100 children** before their 5th birthday.

A history of rotavirus

Before vaccine

Almost all children have had a rotavirus infection by the time they turn 5 years old. Before vaccine, one child in every 100 in Canada was being hospitalized with rotavirus diarrhea. The peak age for rotavirus diarrhea is in infancy, between 6 and 24 months of age.

And while deaths from rotavirus were uncommon in developed countries, they still happened (about 20 to 60 infants died per year in the United States).

After vaccine

In the United States, rotavirus vaccine for infants was introduced in 2006. Within 3 years, the number of young children hospitalized for rotavirus had dropped by 90%. In some areas, yearly outbreaks of rotavirus infection no longer occurred.

And even though older children and adults had not been vaccinated, rotavirus infection dropped in these groups as well, since they usually catch the illness from younger children.

Rotavirus vaccine was first licensed in Canada in 2006 and was recommended for routine use in all babies in 2010. A decrease in hospitalizations for rotavirus gastroenteritis has been observed in several hospitals.

Other countries with routine rotavirus immunization programs, including Australia, Brazil and Mexico, have seen the number of severe rotavirus infections decrease by about 85%.

Studies have shown that rotavirus vaccine also protects children in developing countries. The World Health Organization now recommends that *all* infants receive rotavirus vaccine.

The germ

Rotavirus has two proteins in its outer shell, the G protein and the P protein: both can stimulate production of protective antibodies. There are many different rotavirus strains, but most infections in Canada are caused by six types.

How the germ causes illness

Rotavirus infects and kills cells that line the surface of the small intestine. The body loses fluids and salts, causing large amounts of watery diarrhea. The damage to the intestine also makes it difficult to digest certain foods, especially carbohydrates (found in bread products, fruit, milk, yogurt and many other foods). Bacteria in the large intestine (colon) break down these undigested carbohydrates into small bits, causing even more diarrhea and water loss.

In the first few days after infection, the intestinal lining shrinks, allowing the unaffected parts to fuse together and form a barrier against more fluid loss. By 6 to 10 days after infection, the small intestine is back to normal.

How rotavirus spreads

Rotavirus is highly contagious, both before and after symptoms develop.

Children with rotavirus diarrhea shed a massive number of viruses in stool. After diarrhea resolves, shedding can continue for up to 21 days. Rotavirus survives for a long time on surfaces, and many disinfectants do not destroy it. Virus can spread from an infected to an uninfected child when they touch, or when an uninfected child mouths a contaminated toy or surface that an infected child has touched.

> **Young children spread rotavirus**
> The universal habit in toddlers and young children of putting their fingers as well as toys and other objects in their mouths, ensures that rotavirus will rapid spread quickly in families and in child care settings.

Diaper changing can also spread rotavirus, especially when people are not very careful about hygiene. When changing the diaper of an infected child, a caregiver's hands are contaminated with large amounts of rotavirus. If the caregiver doesn't wash hands and clean the change table thoroughly after diapering, the virus soon spreads to other people, objects and surfaces.

The illness

Symptoms. Illness can begin any time between 18 hours to 3 days after exposure. It begins suddenly with fever and vomiting, followed by diarrhea that lasts 5 to 7 days. Up to 20 bouts of vomiting and 20 episodes of diarrhea can occur in a single day. Some children only experience vomiting.

Rotavirus infections are usually milder in the first 3 months of life, because of protective antibodies that have passed from mother to infant. It's most severe in children aged 3 to 24 months. Most hospitalizations for rotavirus (about 63%) occur in this age group.

Giving fluids is critical. If fluids lost through diarrhea and vomiting are not replaced (through drinking), a child can become dehydrated very quickly. Dehydration is severe when a child loses more than 10% body weight.

Most children with rotavirus infection can be cared for at home with oral rehydration solutions (ORS), which are available at a pharmacy. These

> **Dehydration happens fast**
>
> A baby with rotavirus loses water very quickly, by drinking less, vomiting and having diarrhea. Dehydration can happen as soon as 6 hours after illness starts.

solutions contain water, salts and minerals in concentrations designed to prevent dehydration by replacing what is lost in diarrhea.

Severe cases hospitalized. In a study of 335 Canadian children hospitalized with rotavirus diarrhea, most illnesses lasted 4 to 7 days. These children were severely ill: 94% needed intravenous fluids. Fortunately, just one month after falling ill, almost all were healthy again, and nearly 90% were back to or almost at their pre-infection weight.

Rotavirus can be more severe and last longer in children who have a weakened immune system.

Complications

Severe dehydration can cause shock, with a rapid pulse and drop in blood pressure. If shock is not treated, a child's circulation can fail and he can die.

Long-term effects from rotavirus are rare in Canada. Less than 1% of infected children experience **persistent diarrhea**, vomiting or fever lasting longer than 2 weeks.

Death caused by rotavirus diarrhea is rare in Canada and other developed countries. Unfortunately, in poorer regions of the world, rotavirus diarrhea is a major cause of death in young children. In the poorest countries, about one child in every 100 dies of rotavirus diarrhea before age 5.

Diagnosis

If a child is vomiting, has watery diarrhea and fever, it could be rotavirus, especially if a baby is 6 to 23 months old and has these symptoms in the late winter or early spring.

Rapid tests can find rotavirus in a child's stool.

Treatment

Prevent dehydration. There is no specific treatment for rotavirus infections. Steps to prevent dehydration include maintaining fluid intake:
- Continue to breastfeed. Most babies with rotavirus diarrhea are thirsty and will breastfeed when offered.
- Give oral rehydration solutions (ORS) to replace lost fluids.

If dehydration occurs, a baby may need to have fluids replaced intravenously (through a needle in a vein). This treatment happens in hospital.

Post-recovery

Immunity after rotavirus infection doesn't last long. But once a child has had rotavirus infection, later infections are usually less severe.

The vaccine

Type of vaccine

Two rotavirus vaccines are available in Canada. **RotaTeq (RV5)** was approved for use in 2006 and **Rotarix (RV1)** in 2007.

Both vaccines are very effective.

How rotavirus vaccine is made

Process. RV5 vaccine was created by recombinant gene technology. (Recombinant means "putting genes together", in this case, combining different viruses in the laboratory.)

RV5 vaccine was made by combining genes from human and calf rotaviruses. The vaccine strains contain genes that make proteins on the surface of the human rotavirus, which produce immunity, while the remaining genes come from calf rotavirus. The calf rotavirus is used because it does not cause illness in humans. But when it is modified to make the vaccine, it stimulates the immune system to make protective antibodies against the human rotaviruses. This vaccine contains 5 vaccine strains. Each strain is grown separately in monkey kidney cell cultures, extracted, purified, then combined in one liquid vaccine.

RV1 vaccine contains a single, live attenuated (weakened) human rotavirus strain which produces immunity against several strains. The strain was weakened by growing it repeatedly in monkey kidney cultures. The weakened virus is then produced in monkey kidney cell cultures, extracted and purified.

For general information on vaccine additives, see Chapter 4.

Available forms of rotavirus vaccine

Both rotavirus vaccines are available in liquid form, and are not combined with any other vaccines.

How the vaccine is given

Rotavirus vaccines are given by mouth. If an incomplete dose is given for any reason (e.g., an infant spits or regurgitates the vaccine) a replacement dose does not need to be given.

Schedule of vaccination

RV5 requires 3 doses (*4 to 10 weeks apart*). **RV1** requires 2 doses (*at least* 4 weeks apart). For best results, the first dose is given as soon as possible after an infant is 6 weeks old, and the series is completed as early as possible and no later than age 8 months.

Infants only. The first dose of rotavirus vaccine is given to infants between 6 and 20 weeks of age, and the series completed by age 8 months. The first dose is not given after 20 weeks because there is some concern about a risk of intussusception (a type of bowel blockage) in older infants.

The vaccines are often given to infants at the same time as other routine vaccines: at 2, 4 and 6 months of age (**RV5**), or at 2 and 4 months (**RV1**).

Neither vaccine is recommended for babies over 8 months old because of concern about intussusception (a type of bowel blockage), which is more common in older babies.

Older children and adults do not need rotavirus vaccine because the disease is very mild in these groups.

> **Length of protection isn't known**
> - Rotavirus infections don't produce long-lasting immunity against reinfection: it isn't expected that the vaccines will either. Studies suggest that protection lasts for 2 to 3 years.
> - However, because severe rotavirus illness occurs mainly in children under 2 years old, vaccination *does* help to prevent severe illness.

Possible side effects of rotavirus vaccine

Rare and mild. Infants rarely have side effects from either rotavirus vaccine. One study showed a small increase in cases of mild diarrhea and vomiting after the RV5 vaccine.

Intussusception (bowel blockage) is a rare condition in infants, occurring in about 34 infants per 100,000 per year. A very small risk of intussusception (1 to 5 cases per 100,000 doses) has been noted after rotavirus vaccine in the United States and some other countries.

Reasons to avoid or delay rotavirus vaccine

Immunosuppression (compromised immune system function). Rotavirus vaccine is not given to infants with a serious immune system disorder because it might cause severe diarrhea.

After an infant receives rotavirus vaccine, small quantities of the vaccine virus may be shed in the stool. But it's rare that the vaccine virus transmits to other people. Infants sharing a home with a person who is severely immunosuppressed should still be immunized. The benefits of the vaccine—protecting a child from getting rotavirus and transmitting it to the immunosuppressed person—far outweigh the very small risk of infecting an immunosuppressed family member with the vaccine virus.

This risk can be virtually eliminated by careful handwashing after contact with stool (e.g., after changing diapers).

Intussusception. An infant who has had this type of bowel blockage should not get rotavirus vaccine, in case the condition recurs. Infants born with a gastrointestinal tract malformation (e.g., Meckel's diverticulum) that may contribute to intussusception should not get rotavirus vaccine until the condition is corrected surgically.

Gastroenteritis. Babies with moderate-to-severe gastroenteritis should not get the vaccine until their condition improves, because the vaccine may not work.

Pregnancy. Infants sharing a household with a pregnant woman should be vaccinated. Most women are immune to rotavirus, which in any case is not a serious disease in pregnancy or a risk to the developing fetus.

Breastfed infants should receive the rotavirus vaccine.

For general information on reasons to delay or avoid a vaccine or vaccines, see Chapter 6.

The results of vaccination

Evidence that rotavirus vaccine works:
- Studies showed that rotavirus vaccine prevents about 75% of all rotavirus gastroenteritis infections, and 85% to 98% of severe infections.
- The vaccine may help to protect babies even before they have received all the required doses. One study showed that protection after 2 doses was 81%, and after one dose, 69%.
- Protection may last for up to 3 years (94% against severe rotavirus infection and 63% against any rotavirus infection). A large controlled study in Finland and several Latin American countries showed that RV1 vaccine was 85% effective in preventing severe rotavirus disease in the first year and 83% effective in the first two years after vaccination.

- In the United States, the hospitalization rate for rotavirus infection in children decreased by 50% in the first year after vaccine was introduced, even though only 33% of eligible infants received the vaccine.
- Rotavirus infection is decreasing in all age groups, which means that older children and adults are being protected indirectly while vaccinating infants. The same is true of infants less than 6 weeks months of age, who are too young to be vaccinated.
- In many parts of the United States, rotavirus vaccination has delayed, reduced or even prevented the usual yearly rotavirus outbreaks.
- Rotavirus vaccine is effective in many poorer countries. Protection is less than in developed countries, but in areas with high infant mortality, death rates from diarrhea have been significantly reduced.

Snapshots

- Rotavirus can be a mild illness, but it can also put almost 1% of Canadian children in hospital before their 5th birthday.
- Most children who are hospitalized for gastroenteritis have a rotavirus infection.
- Vaccination is very effective in reducing the risk of severe illness and hospitalization in infants.
- In healthy infants, rotavirus vaccines are very safe and very effective.

21

Rubella

Rubella, also known as "German measles", is caused by a virus. Common symptoms are fever, sore throat, swollen glands and small red spots that last a few days. When children get rubella, it's usually a mild illness. Many don't even get a fever or rash, and sometimes rubella causes no symptoms at all.

In teenagers and adults, rubella can be a more serious disease. When a woman is infected in the first 20 weeks of pregnancy, the virus then infects her fetus. Sometimes, the unborn baby will die. Babies who survive to delivery are likely to have severe disabilities, which could include damage to their brain, eyes, ears, heart and other organs. This is called "congenital rubella syndrome".

A history of rubella

Before vaccine

Women at risk. In North America, outbreaks of rubella used to be common. They occurred almost every spring, mainly in children 6 to 10 years old, with larger epidemics about every 7 years. About 85% of people had rubella by the time they reached age 20. That translated into about 250,000 rubella infections every year in Canada before the vaccine was introduced. The other 15% of people were therefore still "susceptible" to rubella (meaning they were not immune, and therefore at risk of contracting it). The people at greatest risk were women of child-bearing age, who could be infected while pregnant.

Rubella in pregnancy. An eye doctor in Australia first noted the danger of rubella to unborn babies in 1941. Dr. Alan Gregg cared for a number of infants who had been born with cataracts. He discovered that their mothers had all had rubella at an early stage of pregnancy. Other doctors in many parts of the world confirmed his findings. Many of these babies were also deaf or had malformed hearts.

A huge epidemic. During a worldwide rubella epidemic in 1964, there were about 12.5 million cases of rubella in the United States alone. Nearly 30,000 expectant mothers were infected in the first 20 weeks of pregnancy. More than 8,000 babies died and about 20,000 who survived had congenital rubella syndrome. Compare this with an "average" (pre-vaccine) year, when about 2,000 babies were born with congenital rubella syndrome in the United States.

After vaccine

Rubella virus was first isolated and grown in a laboratory in 1962. Three different rubella vaccines were developed and approved for use in 1968–69. Then, as now, the goal of rubella vaccination programs was to prevent congenital rubella syndrome.

At first, the rubella vaccine was used in two different ways, in different countries.

The American strategy. The United States and several Canadian provinces or territories used a three-step program:

1. All children were vaccinated at about 1 year of age.
2. All women of child-bearing age were tested for immunity to rubella.
3. Women whose tests showed they were not immune to rubella (and so at risk of contracting it) were vaccinated before they became pregnant.

The American strategy was designed to stop the spread of rubella by vaccinating *all* children. Stopping the spread of rubella would prevent non-immune pregnant women from being exposed to the virus.

The British strategy. In the other Canadian provinces or territories and in the United Kingdom, the vaccine was recommended only for girls 10 to 12 years of age and non-immune women. The theory was that vaccinating 10- to 12-year-old girls would eventually lead to fewer women being susceptible to rubella in pregnancy.

But only about 85% of schoolgirls actually received the rubella vaccine, so the plan was not as effective as hoped.

A clear winner. The rate of congenital rubella syndrome in the United Kingdom and in the Canadian provinces or territories using the British plan did not fall as much or as rapidly as in the United States and in the provinces or territories using the American strategy. In 1983, a review led to the adoption across Canada of the American strategy of rubella vaccination for all infants. The United Kingdom also adopted this strategy about 5 years later.

Today, success. The last major epidemic of rubella in North America was in 1965. Since starting routine infant rubella vaccination in 1980, the number of babies born in Canada with congenital rubella syndrome has declined from an estimated 200 per year to an average of 3: a drop of 98.5%. With rare exceptions, these cases have been in babies whose mothers never had either the disease or the vaccine before becoming pregnant.

There are still pockets of rubella in Africa, Europe and other areas of the world—even in Canada!—where routine immunization against rubella is less than 90%. In these places, pregnant women may still be vulnerable to infection.

A rubella outbreak can happen in Canada

In southwestern Ontario in 2005, there were 309 confirmed cases of rubella in a community that opposed vaccination for philosophical reasons. Nearly 200 cases were in unimmunized children 5 to 14 years of age, and 10 were in pregnant women. Fortunately, no cases of congenital rubella were reported. And because immunization rates in Canada are generally high, this outbreak did not spread.

The germ

Rubella virus only infects humans.

How the germ causes illness

When a person inhales droplets containing rubella viruses, these germs infect cells lining the nose and throat, then spread to lymph glands in the neck. After about 2 weeks, the virus enters the bloodstream, spreading to the skin, eyes, respiratory tract and other organs. A rash appears at the peak of infection but is also a sign that recovery has begun.

During pregnancy. Rubella virus in the bloodstream during pregnancy can infect the placenta, then the fetus. Being infected in the womb is completely different from rubella infection after birth. With congenital rubella syndrome, cells of the embryo and developing fetus are unable to get rid of the virus. When these fetal cells are infected, cells can't divide as they normally would. The infection interrupts growth and development in many organs, causing damage to the unborn baby.

How rubella spreads

Spread of rubella virus requires close contact between people. An infected person's cough or sneeze spreads droplets containing many virus particles to the nose or throat of another person.

The period of time that a person with rubella can spread it to others lasts from about 7 days *before* the start of the rash to at least 4 days *after* the rash appears. As for mumps, measles and chickenpox, this infection can spread *before* an infected person is diagnosed.

Rubella is *most* contagious a few days before and after the rash appears.

Babies with congenital rubella syndrome are contagious for a longer time: they may release rubella virus in their saliva and urine for more than a year.

Rubella is less contagious than measles or chickenpox. Before vaccination, about 85% of children got rubella compared with over 95% who caught measles and chickenpox.

The illness

Symptoms. The incubation period for rubella, meaning the time between exposure to the virus and the start of symptoms, can be long: anywhere from 14 to 21 days. No symptoms occur in the first week after exposure. Lymph glands may swell in the second week, especially behind the ears and at the back of the head.

By the end of week two, a mild illness begins, with low-grade fever, aches and pains, and red eyes. Rash usually appears after 1 or 2 days of mild illness. If the lymph glands didn't enlarge earlier, they are likely to swell with the start of other symptoms.

Rash. Small red spots appear first on the face and scalp, then spread rapidly down the body. They begin to fade within 1 to 3 days. The rubella rash is very similar to rashes caused by many other viral infections, making rubella difficult to diagnose from the rash alone.

Severity depends on age and stage
- In children, rubella is usually a mild illness. Many don't get sick at all or are mildly ill without rash. They can spread the infection to others.
- Teenagers and adults are much more likely to have symptoms and may also have complications, such as joint pain.
- Woman who are pregnant and not immune are at highest risk. Rubella can cause fetal malformations or miscarriage if a woman is infected in the first 20 weeks of pregnancy.

Complications

Joint pain. The most common complication of rubella is joint pain, which happens more often in adults and especially in women (50% to 70%) than in children. Most women who experience joint pain after rubella infection do not have arthritis (i.e., there is no redness, swelling or limitation of movement). The pain lasts a few days to a few weeks and almost always clears completely.

Rarely, a person develops chronic arthritis after rubella. It is not clear whether rubella virus causes the arthritis, triggers an underlying joint disease or is completely unrelated to chronic joint problems.

Other complications of rubella infection are uncommon. A very few children develop **thrombocytopenia**, a condition that lowers, temporarily, the number of platelets in blood (particles that help with blood clot formation). Small hemorrhages and bruises show up in the skin. Although this condition is rare, it can cause major problems, especially if there is bleeding into the brain. Usually, the platelet problem goes away when infection resolves.

Encephalitis (inflammation of the brain) occurs in about 1 in 6,000 cases of rubella. It is more common in adults than in children. Encephalitis in rubella cases is the result of an allergic-type reaction to the presence of the virus. The virus does not invade the brain cells, as in most other types of encephalitis. Symptoms disappear over time. It is uncommon for rubella to cause permanent brain damage.

SSPE. Rubella can cause another, very different kind of encephalitis, called SSPE (subacute sclerosing panencephalitis). Most cases of SSPE are caused by measles, but it can also be caused by chronic infection of brain cells with rubella virus. Most cases of SSPE occur in children with congenital rubella syndrome and begin years after the actual rubella infection.

SSPE caused by rubella is no different than SSPE caused by measles. The immune system attacks infected cells and destroys nerve cells in the brain. The affected person experiences progressive deterioration: changes in personality and behaviour, intellectual impairment, seizures and coma. There is no cure for SSPE, although some drugs may slow the rate of deterioration. **SSPE is always fatal**.

Congenital rubella syndrome

If a woman is infected with rubella in the first 20 weeks of her pregnancy, chances are high (more than 8 in 10) that the fetus will also be infected. A baby who survives to delivery will likely have congenital rubella syndrome.

With **congenital rubella syndrome**, infection causes two types of abnormalities:
- It interferes with fetal cell division, so that organs such as the brain, heart, eyes and ears become malformed.
- Other organs are affected because the virus kills cells directly, causing inflammation in the liver, spleen and bone marrow.

When a woman becomes infected determines the degree of damage to the fetus. If infection occurs in the first 12 weeks of pregnancy, the baby is usually born with multiple disabilities (see Table 21.1). If infection occurs between 16 and 20 weeks, deafness is usually the only complication. Infection after 20 weeks of pregnancy does not affect the fetus.

In about one of 5 fetal infections, the damage is so severe that the fetus dies and the woman has a miscarriage. One out of every 10 infected babies dies of complications in the first 12 months of life.

Table 21.1
Malformations associated with congenital rubella syndrome

Body part affected	Resulting abnormality
General	Low birth weight, impaired growth
Brain	Abnormally small brain, severe developmental delay, autism, SSPE
Eyes	Cataracts, absent or small eyes, glaucoma, blindness
Ears	Deafness
Heart	Malformation
Liver	Hepatitis
Bone marrow	Low platelet count causing bleeding
Lungs	Chronic pneumonia
Pancreas	Diabetes
Thyroid	Hypothyroidism

Diagnosis

A blood test is needed. Many viral infections cause an illness identical to rubella, right down to the type of rash. A blood test to detect elevations in antibody to rubella is needed to accurately diagnosis it. Tests to detect rubella virus in the throat, blood or urine are available in some laboratories.

Treatment

There is no specific treatment for rubella. Symptoms (such as headache, aches and pains, and joint pain) can be relieved with acetaminophen (e.g., Tempra, Tylenol). The damage associated with congenital rubella syndrome is irreversible.

Post-recovery

Immunity following rubella usually last for life, though rare cases of reinfection have been reported. One exception is children with congenital rubella syndrome, who are often unable to develop immunity to the virus and may redevelop rubella if they are exposed.

The vaccine

Type of vaccine

Live attenuated virus vaccine. Rubella vaccine is a live virus vaccine that has been attenuated (weakened). This means that the vaccine contains a live virus that multiplies in the body after it is given by injection, but it does not cause rubella. Rather, it acts like natural infection: the virus infects, multiplies and stimulates immunity.

The vaccine virus does not cause any illness in most people (see "Possible side effects of rubella vaccine", below).

How rubella vaccine is made

Producing weakened strains. The vaccine strain used in Canada, the United States and all other countries with immunization programs except for Japan, is called "the RA27/3 vaccine". This strain was isolated and then weakened by repeatedly growing it in human cell cultures.

Process. The virus is grown in cell culture, then extracted and purified. It is combined with measles and mumps vaccines (as MMR) or with measles, mumps and varicella vaccines (as MMRV vaccine), and freeze-dried.

For general information on vaccine additives, see Chapter 4.

Available forms of rubella vaccine

Combinations. Rubella vaccine is only available in Canada in combination with measles and mumps (MMR) or with measles, mumps and varicella (MMRV) vaccines. It is not available as a single vaccine in Canada.

Vaccines for children, adolescents and adults. The same MMR vaccines and dosage are used for all age groups.

MMRV is not recommended for individuals over 12 years of age because it has not yet been tested in older children and adults.

How the vaccine is given

The freeze-dried combination MMR or MMRV is mixed with sterile distilled water and is usually given as a single injection beneath the skin. The MMRV vaccine and one brand of the MMR vaccine may also be injected into muscle.

For more information, see "Getting the Shot" in Chapter 4.

Schedule of vaccination

Infants and children (under age 7). Young children in Canada receive 2 doses of MMR or MMRV vaccine. The first dose is at 12 to 15 months of age. The second is at age 18 months in some provinces and territories, and later in others. The second dose must be given, at the latest, before school entry (at 4 to 6 years of age). Both schedules are effective.

Children and adolescents (7 to 17 years of age). Older children and teens *not* previously immunized should get at least one dose of a vaccine containing rubella. However, if they need measles or mumps vaccine as well, they may be given 2 doses of MMR or MMRV.
- MMR or MMRV may be used in children up to 12 years of age.
- Anyone over 12 years old should get MMR.

MMR doses should be *at least* 4 weeks apart and MMRV doses *at least* 6 weeks apart.

Adults who, when tested, show no evidence of having received vaccine or having had rubella should get one dose.

Women. All women of child-bearing age need a blood test for immunity to rubella, preferably before their first pregnancy.
- *If a woman isn't pregnant* and her blood shows no antibody to rubella, she should be immunized with MMR to prevent infection with rubella. To allow immunity to develop, she should avoid becoming pregnant for one month after vaccination for rubella.
- *If she is already pregnant* and testing shows no antibody to rubella, vaccination should be delayed until after delivery. Ideally, the

vaccine should be given before leaving the hospital. Otherwise, it may be forgotten.

Boosters (to enhance prior vaccinations). Boosters are not needed by anyone who has received at least one dose of a vaccine containing rubella (MMR or MMRV).

Long-lasting protection. The immune response to rubella vaccine is very similar to the response after rubella infection. Studies show that protection lasts for more than 20 years.

Preventing congenital rubella syndrome: Priorities

- Adolescent and adult women:
  - All women of child-bearing age should be assessed for immunity to rubella
  - Those who are not immune should be vaccinated as soon as possible (at least one month before pregnancy)
  - Those who are already pregnant should be vaccinated just after delivery (ideally, before leaving hospital)
  - Young immigrant and refugee women are often not immune and should be assessed as soon as possible after entry to Canada.
- Non-immune women at high risk of being exposed to rubella (e.g., in educational or health care settings)
- Non-immune people who work with children
- Non-immune health care workers
- Non-immune travellers to communities or areas of the world where rubella commonly occurs

---

Possible side effects of rubella vaccine

Mild. Infants rarely have any side effects after rubella vaccine. A few young children develop mild fever and rash. Both the frequency and seriousness of side effects after rubella vaccination increase with age, as does severity of the disease.

Joint pain. The most common side effect of rubella vaccine is painful joints, usually in the knees and fingers. This affects adults much more often than children. About 1 in 7 adult women have some joint pain following vaccination, compared with fewer than 1 in 100 children.

Arthritis (joint pain plus inflammation—redness, swelling and tenderness) is rare.

Thrombocytopenia. This condition is rare, but a few children (one case per 30–40,000 doses) develop thrombocytopenia (low platelets in the blood) after rubella vaccination (see *Complications*).

For information on possible side effects after receiving a combination vaccine, see Chapter 6, Adverse events and common concerns.

> **Complications of infection happen much more often than side effects from vaccine**
>
> - Adults, especially women, are more likely to experience **joint pain**, and to have more severe pain, following rubella infection than following rubella vaccine.
> - Although the condition is rare, the risk of **thrombocytopenia** is higher with rubella infection than after rubella vaccination.

Reasons to avoid or delay rubella vaccine

Immunosuppression (compromised immune system function). As with all live vaccines, rubella vaccine is not given to people with a serious immune system disorder caused by disease or certain medications.

For more information, see Chapter 3, When extra protection is needed.

During pregnancy. Rubella vaccine is not given in pregnancy because of a *theoretical risk* of transmitting the vaccine virus to the fetus. But there is *no evidence that rubella vaccine can harm the fetus*. There have been no cases of congenital rubella syndrome in several thousand infants born to women who received rubella vaccine just before or during pregnancy. Ideally, a woman who needs to be immunized should delay pregnancy by 4 weeks following vaccination with MMR. But if the vaccine was given before she knew she is pregnant, there is *no need for concern* or for the pregnancy to be terminated.

A pregnant woman's other children should be vaccinated according to the routine schedule. The virus contained in the rubella vaccine does not spread from person to person.

Recent injection with immune globulin (IG) or other blood products. IG and other blood products may contain antibody to rubella virus that will interfere with vaccine effectiveness. Vaccination must be delayed for 3 to 11 months, depending on the type and dosage of IG or other blood product used.

For general information on reasons to delay or avoid a vaccine or vaccines, see Chapter 6.

The results of vaccination

Evidence that rubella vaccine works:
- Controlled studies have shown that over 95% of people vaccinated with MMR or MMRV are protected against rubella. For most, vaccination means long-lasting, if not life-long, immunity from this disease.
- There have been no reports of congenital rubella syndrome acquired in Canada since 2000. The few cases that have occurred in recent years were in women who had been infected in other countries.

Snapshots

- Rubella is not a serious illness in children. But when a woman is infected with rubella in pregnancy, her unborn baby may die or suffer permanent damage.
- Outbreaks of rubella still occur in Canada, in groups who have not been immunized. In 2005, more than 300 cases were reported in southwestern Ontario. But because immunization levels are generally high, the disease did not spread outside this area.
- Rubella vaccine is safe, effective and causes no serious reactions in children.

- The routine immunization of children in Canada has reduced the occurrence of congenital rubella syndrome to an average of 3 cases per year.
- All children should be vaccinated against rubella in an effort to eradicate rubella virus and congenital rubella syndrome.
- All women of child-bearing age need a blood test to determine their immunity to rubella, especially if they are planning pregnancy. When a woman is not immune, she should be vaccinated, ideally before becoming pregnant.
- All pregnant women in Canada are tested for immunity to rubella. When found to be non-immune, they should be vaccinated as soon as possible after the birth of their child and preferably, before leaving hospital.

22

Tetanus

Tetanus is a disease caused by a toxin (poison), which is made by bacteria called *Clostridium tetani*. The toxin blocks normal control of nerve reflexes in the spinal cord, causing muscles throughout the body to contract or spasm. These contractions last a long time and are very painful. They can interfere with breathing and cause death. Tetanus is sometimes called "lockjaw" because a person's jaws clench very tightly when jaw muscles spasm.

Tetanus bacteria can form spores, which are seed-like cells with an external coat that protects them in the environment. Tetanus spores survive for many years outside the body and are common not only in dirt but also in dust—even dust in hospitals! Anyone, anywhere, who is not vaccinated and does not have antibody to tetanus can contract the disease.

A history of tetanus

Before vaccine

The bacteria that cause tetanus were identified in 1890, and the fact that they produce a toxin that causes the disease was discovered a year later.

Before tetanus vaccination became routine in the 1940s, there were 60 to 75 cases (including 40 to 50 deaths) each year in Canada. Tetanus has always been more common in males than in females. Most cases of tetanus involved newborns, but the bacteria also affected older boys and young men. During wars, tetanus killed many wounded soldiers.

The development of tetanus antitoxin (which is different from the vaccine) made it possible to neutralize the effect of tetanus toxin. Treatment with antitoxin, combined with improved wound care, led to a decline in the number of tetanus cases and deaths after 1920 in Canada, the United States and other industrialized countries.

In countries that do not vaccinate against tetanus, this disease still kills. Newborn infants can get tetanus through infection of the stump of the umbilical cord. In 2012, an estimated 61,000 newborns around the world died of tetanus.

After vaccine

Tetanus toxoid, the vaccine against tetanus, became available in Canada and the United States in 1938. Its routine use during World War II lowered the rate of tetanus among wounded soldiers in American and British forces by over 30 times compared with World War I.

The success of tetanus toxoid in wartime led to the recommendation, in 1944, of routine immunization for all children in Canada and the United States for the following reasons:
• Tetanus spores are everywhere in the environment.
• The death rate from tetanus, at 10% to 20% even with treatment, is high.
• The vaccine was safe and effective.

The number of tetanus cases has declined dramatically in countries with programs to vaccinate all infants. Over the past 15 years in Canada, annual numbers of cases ranged from 1 to 6 cases, with an average of 4 per year.

The germ

Tetanus germs exist in two forms: as growing bacteria and spores. Tetanus bacteria live and grow in the large intestine of humans and many animals, including horses, dogs, guinea pigs, sheep and cattle. The tetanus germ is anaerobic, which means that it only grows where there is little or no oxygen. The bacteria produce spores as they grow in the intestines. These spores are excreted in feces, contaminating the environment.

Tetanus spores are covered with a tough coating that allows them to survive outside the body of humans or animals. The spores cannot be killed by boiling or by most disinfectants. They do not multiply but they are able to stay alive in soil and dust for many years.

Tetanus bacteria will always be with us

Tetanus bacteria can never be eradicated from the environment. Studies have shown that almost one-third of soil samples collected in North America contain tetanus spores. Spores have also been found in street dust as well as in dust in houses and hospitals.

How the germ causes illness

The disease begins when spores from dirt or dust get into tissue beneath the skin through an injury, usually a puncture, cut or bite. The severity of injury doesn't matter—tetanus can happen after minor injuries that don't require medical attention, such as a scrape or bite. Puncture wounds (e.g., stepping on a nail or being poked by a thorn while gardening), have a higher risk of tetanus compared with cuts, because these wounds can be difficult to clean thoroughly.

Once inside tissue, tetanus spores can change into growing bacteria if the amount of oxygen in the wound is low (i.e., when the wound is not cleaned properly and damaged or dead tissue is not removed). As the bacteria grow, they release toxin into the tissue.

> **?** **Did you know?**
> Tetanus toxin is a nerve poison. It is one of the most powerful poisons in nature.

The smallest dose of tetanus toxin will kill an adult: less than 2 ng (2 nanograms is less than 2 billionth of a gram, or 0.000000002 g). The toxin reaches the spinal cord through the bloodstream and by travelling up nerves from muscle. Once there, it blocks the activity of certain nerve cells and normal control of spinal reflexes is lost. This loss of control causes excess stimulation of muscles throughout the body. Muscles contract uncontrollably, causing severe pain.

How tetanus spreads

Spores. Of all the vaccine-preventable diseases, tetanus is unique because it is not contagious, meaning it does not spread from person to person. Infection only happens when spores in the environment get under the skin as a result of injury.

The illness

Incubation varies. Most tetanus cases begin within 1 to 7 days of injury. Rarely, symptoms have been delayed for up to 60 days after injury.

Symptoms. Muscle spasms, which can be triggered by a sudden noise or movement, are prolonged, uncontrollable and painful. The first spasms are usually of the jaw muscles, making swallowing very difficult, followed by spasms of the muscles of the face, neck, chest, abdomen, arms and legs. All muscles can go into spasm at the same time. The person with tetanus is awake and alert despite repeated spasms. The spasms are frequent and intense for 1 to 4 weeks, then gradually subside.

Complications

Tetanus is a severe disease. The death rate varies from 10% to over 80% and is highest in infants and the elderly. Even with treatment in a modern intensive care unit, the death rate is 10% to 20%. In poor or under-resourced parts of the world that lack adequate health and sanitation facilities, death rates are much higher, especially in newborn infants.

Suffocation. A muscle spasm of the vocal cords can cause immediate death by blocking the airway.

Other complications of tetanus may include:
• Choking spells due to difficulty swallowing
• Bone fractures from severe muscle spasms
• Weight loss because a person can't eat
• Problems associated with any severe prolonged illness requiring intensive care, such as pneumonia (infection of the lungs) and skin ulcers
• Lasting difficulties with speech, memory and mental function.

Diagnosis

The diagnosis of tetanus is based on typical muscle spasms developing within days of an injury. Bacteria can sometimes be identified in a culture from an infected wound. Often tetanus bacteria are not found because so few are needed to cause illness.

Treatment

Treatment of tetanus involves:
• Surgical cleaning of the wound and removing dead tissue that might contain spores
• Killing tetanus bacteria in the wound with antibiotics to prevent them from producing more toxin
• Neutralizing toxin in the wound and blood with tetanus immune globulin (antitoxin) to prevent it from binding to nerve cells
• Relieving and preventing muscle spasms with drugs.

Tetanus immune globulin (antitoxin or TIG), is made from blood donated by adult volunteers who have been vaccinated repeatedly with tetanus toxoid. They develop high concentrations of antibodies to tetanus toxin. Plasma (the liquid part of blood) is extracted and partially purified to concentrate the antibodies.

Volunteers are tested to make sure they are not infected with HIV, hepatitis B, hepatitis C or other blood-borne viruses. No infections with these viruses have occurred as the result of using TIG.

TIG is given by injection into muscle.

Post-recovery

Such a small amount of toxin is released during the course of the disease that survivors usually do not develop immunity to tetanus. There have been recurrent cases. Therefore, all survivors need to be fully immunized to protect them in future.

The vaccine

Type of vaccine

Inactivated bacterial toxin. The vaccine against tetanus, known as "tetanus toxoid", is an inactivated bacterial toxin. Treating the tetanus toxin with formaldehyde makes the toxin harmless without affecting its ability to induce antibody. Antibodies can neutralize the toxin and prevent it from binding to nerve cells.

How tetanus toxoid is made

Process. Tetanus bacteria are grown in liquid culture, releasing toxin as they multiply. The bacteria are removed by filtering, the toxin is purified from the fluid, then concentrated and treated with formaldehyde to turn it into a harmless toxoid. The final vaccine contains less than 0.02% (less than 200 parts per million) of residual formaldehyde.

For general information on vaccine additives, see Chapter 4.

Available forms of tetanus toxoid

A combined vaccine. In Canada, tetanus toxoid is only available in combination with one or more other vaccines. For more information, see "Vaccine types" in Chapter 4.

How the vaccine is given

Tetanus vaccines are given by injection into muscle. For more information, see "Getting the Shot" in Chapter 4.

Schedule of vaccination

Infants and children (under age 7). For routine immunization of young children in Canada, 4 doses of tetanus vaccine (in combination with other vaccines) are given at 2, 4, 6 and 18 months. A booster dose follows at 4 to 6 years of age. If a dose is missed or delayed for any reason, the missing dose should be given but the series does not have to be started again.

Children (age 7 and over) adolescents and adults. For this group, whether as an initial vaccine or as a booster, a combination of tetanus toxoid, lower-dose diphtheria toxoid, and the adult form of acellular pertussis vaccine is used.

An adolescent booster is given routinely to teens (at 14 to 16 years of age).

Adult boosters. Tetanus toxoid does not provide lifelong immunity. A booster every 10 years is recommended.

Did you know?

Many adults do not get their booster shots for tetanus. They should receive *at least* one booster at age 50, and a booster dose every 10 years if they are at higher risk of wounds contaminated with soil (e.g., gardeners, farmers or members of the military).

Preventing tetanus infection post-exposure

People who have a contaminated injury need a tetanus booster if they had their last dose more than 10 years before (for minor wounds) or more than 5 years before (for more extensive wounds). Individuals who have not had 3 doses of vaccine, or whose immune system does not work well, must also receive tetanus immuneglobulin (TIG).

Possible side effects of tetanus toxoid

Tetanus toxoid is very safe.

Local reactions. Redness, swelling, pain and tenderness at the injection site are the most common reactions. The likelihood of a local reaction increases with the number of doses received. Most people have a local reaction after getting a booster shot.

Severe local reactions (extensive swelling, redness and pain) occur in less than 2% of people who get a booster, and usually in adults who have received boosters too often (i.e., more than once every 10 years). While pain and tenderness may limit mobility of the arm for a few days, these reactions cause no permanent damage.

Other mild reactions following tetanus vaccination may include fever, chills, headache, fatigue and muscle aches.

For information on possible side effects after receiving a combination vaccine, see Chapter 6, Adverse events and common concerns.

Reasons to delay or avoid tetanus vaccine

For general information on reasons to delay or avoid a vaccine or vaccines, see Chapter 6.

The results of vaccination

Tetanus is extremely rare in people whose immunizations are up-to-date. The only paediatric cases in the United States over the past 20 years have been in children who were not vaccinated because their parents refused immunization. Two children have developed tetanus in Canada since 1991, most recently in 2007.

It is clear from experience with massive programs to protect soldiers in the battlefield and newborns in underdeveloped countries that tetanus toxoid is highly effective.

Evidence that tetanus toxoid works:
- Tetanus has virtually disappeared in countries where the vaccination of infants and children is routine.
- Tetanus is extremely rare in people who are fully immunized.
- Controlled studies show a marked decline in tetanus in newborns if their mothers are vaccinated in pregnancy.

Snapshots

- Tetanus toxoid is one of the safest and most effective vaccines.
- Tetanus is not contagious: it does not spread from person to person. Infection happens when bacterial spores in the environment enter the body through a wound.
- Because tetanus spores are everywhere, the only effective way to prevent tetanus is by vaccination.
- The vaccine prevents the *disease* caused by tetanus toxin. But vaccination can never make tetanus bacteria in the environment disappear.
- Immunity to tetanus decreases with age. Adults need booster doses to be fully protected.
- In countries that do not vaccinate against tetanus, this disease still kills.

III

To find out more

23

Resources

The Internet offers access to a wealth of information about vaccines, diseases and immunization. But it's also a source of misinformation. No one regulates the validity of information that is available to millions of people. It's up to consumers themselves to do this.

Evaluating online information may seem like a daunting task but checking for a few key features can almost always help you determine whether a source is credible and whether the information on offer is reliable. First, this chapter will help you decide if an internet or other resource is worthy of your time and trust.

Later, you'll find the best immunization resources to consult if you're looking for answers to questions or wanting to know more about what you have read in this book.

Tips for evaluating information

In your search for information about vaccines, you will probably come across sources you're not sure about. The questions below can help you judge whether or not information is reliable. These questions were written specifically for online information, but they can be asked about any media source: videos, newspapers, magazines, radio, tabloids, pamphlets or books.

1. What is the source?
- The website should clearly identify the person or organization that produced it.
- The website should give information about the owner of the site and a way to contact the information provider(s).
- The website should be endorsed by a health agency or association that you trust.
- Information from local, regional, national or international organizations may be more reliable than the views of a single person.

2. Is the website up-to-date?
- There should be a date indicating when information was last revised. It should be current.

3. Has the information been reviewed by scientific experts?
- The experts should be identified, with their credentials (degrees, positions, etc.).

4. Is there scientific evidence to support their claims?
- The site should provide references to sources for scientific evidence, such as medical journals or texts, or include actual reports or statistics.

Not all online health information is accurate. Be cautious when you evaluate health information on the Internet, especially if the site:
- Is selling something
- Includes outdated information

- Does not have a clear source identified, or a way to reach someone associated with the site
- Makes unrealistic claims for what a product can do (i.e., they sound too good to be true!)

Ask 5 key questions

If you're visiting a health website for the first time, asking these questions can help you decide whether the site is a credible resource.

- **Who** runs the website? Can you trust them?
- **What** does the site say? Do its claims seem reasonable?
- **When** was the information posted or reviewed? Is it up-to-date?
- **Where** did the information come from? Is it based on scientific research?
- **Why** does the site exist? Is it selling something?

For more information on assessing immunization information on the Internet, see these resources:

Canadian Paediatric Society (CPS), A parent's guide to immunization information on the Internet: www.caringforkids.cps.ca/handouts/immunization_information_on_the_internet

Immunize Canada, Immunization information on the Internet: Can you trust what you read?: http://resources.cpha.ca/immunize.ca/data/0288e.pdf

National Center for Complementary and Integrative Health (U.S. Department of Health and Human Services). Finding and evaluating online resources on complementary health approaches: http://nccam.nih.gov/health/webresources

Identifying anti-vaccination websites

Several studies analyzing websites that oppose vaccination found that they have many features in common:

- They made the same false claims about vaccines.
- They all had links to other anti-vaccination sites.
- Many promote alternative systems of health care—such as homeopathy, naturopathy and chiropractic—as being superior to vaccination.
- More than half provided stories about children who had allegedly been damaged by vaccines.
- Parents were the main source for the stories about the alleged dangers of vaccines.

Anti-vaccine activists also use some common tactics:
- Skewing the evidence (usually by denying or rejecting science that does not support their beliefs).
- Equating anecdotes with evidence.
- Frequently proposing new theories for vaccine harm
- Censorship (by suppressing dissenting opinion or trying to shut down critics).
- Attacking their critics using insults and lawsuits.

In addition to the many false claims already discussed in this book, anti-vaccination websites often imply that:
- Vaccine manufacturers and/or government regulators deliberately under-report adverse reactions (by "covering up" the "truth" about such events).
- Vaccine policy is motivated by profit (e.g., by claiming that manufacturers make enormous profits on vaccines, which influences vaccine recommendations and promotes "cover-up" of reactions).

They are also likely to claim that homeopathy, naturopathy, and alternative medicines enhance immunity better than vaccines.

If you are in doubt...

...about any information you read or hear, don't hesitate to discuss it with a health care professional.

Credible sites and resources

Canadian sites

Canadian Immunization Guide
www.phac-aspc.gc.ca/publicat/cig-gci/index-eng.php

An online "evergreen" version of the *Canadian Immunization Guide* is available here. This document for health care providers is produced by the National Advisory Committee on Immunization and presents recommendations for vaccines used in Canada.

Caring for Kids
www.caringforkids.cps.ca

The Canadian Paediatric Society (CPS) website for parents and caregivers has evidence-based, current, easy-to-read information on vaccines, immunization and a wide range of other child and youth health topics, developed with and reviewed by paediatricians.

Canadian Paediatric Society
www.cps.ca

The main CPS website has position statements from the Infectious Diseases and Immunization Committee, written for health care professionals and others who want detailed, scientific information on vaccines and vaccine-preventable diseases.

Information on IMPACT, the vaccine surveillance program, and the Canadian Paediatric Surveillance Program, which helps to monitor rare diseases, is also available here. (For more information, see "Ensuring vaccine safety" in Chapter 5.)

Caring for Kids New to Canada
www.kidsnewtocanada.ca

This CPS-produced website on immigrant and refugee health care highlights many aspects of culturally competent care, including vaccines, travel precautions and specific infectious diseases. See especially "Immunizations: Getting the newcomer child or youth up-to-date".

Immunize Canada
www.immunize.cpha.ca

Managed by the Canadian Public Health Association, Immunize Canada is a coalition of professional and user groups that promotes understanding and use of vaccines in Canada. The goal of Immunize Canada is to help control vaccine-preventable diseases by raising awareness of the benefits and risks of immunization.

Public Health Agency of Canada
www.phac-aspc.gc.ca/im/index-eng.php

This government website has complete, current and credible information for families and health professionals on vaccines and the diseases they prevent.

Two booklets for families are available online and in print: "A parent's guide to vaccination", and "Don't wait, vaccinate! A guide to immunization for First Nations parents and caregivers".

National Advisory Committee on Immunization
www.phac-aspc.gc.ca/naci-ccni/index-eng.php

In addition to the *Canadian Immunization Guide*, new and updated committee recommendations on vaccines and vaccine issues are available here.

The Committee to Advise on Tropical Medicine and Travel (CATMAT)
www.phac-aspc.gc.ca/tmp-pmv/catmat-ccmtmv/index-eng.php

CATMAT is an expert group that provides information for health care providers on health issues related to travel.

Meningitis Research Foundation of Canada
www.meningitis.ca

This website, founded by the parent of a child who died of meningitis, features disease- and vaccine-specific information for families.

American sites

American Academy of Pediatrics
www2.aap.org/immunization
> This section of the American Academy of Pediatrics (AAP) website includes the organization's policy statements on immunization, with information for health care providers on a huge range vaccine-related issues.

Childhood Immunization Support Program
www2.aap.org/immunization/about/programfacts.html
> Founded by the AAP, in partnership with the Centers for Disease Control and Prevention, the Childhood Immunization Support Program has education and resources for parents and paediatricians on immunization issues.

Centers for Disease Control and Prevention
www.cdc.gov
> The Centers for Disease Control and Prevention (CDC) is the federal public health agency in the United States. You can search their massive website using a search engine or an alphabetical menu of health topics.
>
> The CDC's vaccine sub-site (www.cdc.gov/vaccines) has many resources for families, including a booklet called "Parents' Guide to Childhood Immunization", with straightforward information on vaccine-preventable diseases (www.cdc.gov/vaccines/pubs/parents-guide/default.htm).
>
> Other useful features include current U.S. immunization schedules, recommendations from the Advisory Committee on Immunization Practices of the U.S. Public Health Services, vaccine information sheets for parents, information on vaccine safety, instructions on how to report vaccine-related side effects, and a list of reliable resources.

Immunization Action Coalition
www.immunize.org
> This non-profit group of immunization experts works with the CDC to provide health care professionals and the public with the latest immuni-

zation information and accurate, reliable educational materials. Useful information for parents includes personal accounts of people affected by vaccine-preventable diseases, and links to quality resources.

Institute of Medicine
www.iom.edu

A branch of the National Academy of Sciences, the Institute of Medicine (IOM) is an independent, non-profit organization working outside of government to provide unbiased and authoritative advice to decision-makers and the public. They assess the scientific information available on issues of concern, including several reports online related to vaccines.

National Network for Immunization Information
www.immunizationinfo.org

A collaboration of several medical organizations, including the Infectious Diseases Society of America, the Pediatric Infectious Diseases Society and the American Academy of Pediatrics, the National Network for Immunization Information (NNii) publishes "Newsbriefs" each week. They can be received as an e-newsletter and highlight vaccine issues in the news. The site has a searchable database on vaccine-preventable diseases, information on vaccine development and safety, guidelines on evaluating online information, and an annotated list of quality websites.

Parents of Kids with Infectious Diseases
www.pkids.org

This site, known as PKIDS, contains information, articles, and an "Ask the Experts" feature that allows users to e-mail their questions.

Vaccine Education Center at the Children's Hospital of Philadelphia
www.chop.edu/service/vaccine-education-center

This site provides vaccine information for parents and health professionals with focus on vaccine safety, how vaccines work, how they are made, who recommends them, when they should be given, and why they are necessary.

International

World Health Organization
- Immunization
  www.who.int/topics/immunization/en
  The WHO website offers a wealth of authoritative information on immunization and diseases from a global perspective.
- Vaccine Safety Net
  www.who.int/vaccine_safety/initiative/communication/ network/vaccine_safety_websites/en/
  Information from the WHO on vaccine safety and how it is monitored worldwide.
- If you choose not to vaccinate your child, Understand the risks and responsibilities
  www.euro.who.int/__data/assets/pdf_file/0004/160753/If-You-Choose-Not-to-Vaccinate.pdf
  A document for parents.

Vaccine Resource Library
www.path.org/vaccineresources/about.php
  This partnership among U.S. and international groups offers a wide variety of quality, scientifically accurate documents and links to resources on immunization topics.

Books

Offit, Paul A. and Moser, Charlotte A. *Vaccines and Your Child: Separating Fact from Fiction.* New York, N.Y.: Columbia University Press, 2011.

Pickering, Larry K., Baker, C.J., Kimberlin, D.W. and Long, S.S., eds. *Red Book: 2012 Report of the Committee on Infectious Diseases.* Elk Grove Village, IL: American Academy of Pediatrics, 2012.

  This authoritative reference is revised every 3 years.

Plotkin, Stanley A, Orenstein Walter A. and Offit, Paul A. eds. *Vaccines,* 6th edition. Philadelphia, PA: Elsevier Inc., 2013.

Appendix

Vaccines for foreign travel: Details

Some travel-related infections, such as hepatitis A, meningococcus and typhoid, are more likely to occur in children than in adults. Yellow fever vaccine is required for entry into certain countries. These four vaccines will be addressed first.

Hepatitis A vaccine

Hepatitis A is the most common vaccine-preventable infection in travellers. Hepatitis A vaccine is strongly recommended for all people travelling to less developed countries, especially to rural areas or places where adequate sanitation or safe water and food are not always available.

Protective antibodies are already present within 2 weeks of vaccination. And because hepatitis A infection has a long incubation period (2 to

7 weeks), travellers can receive this vaccine up to their day of departure and still have some protection.

For travellers who need both hepatitis A and hepatitis B vaccines, a combined vaccine is available.

Although hepatitis A vaccine is licensed only for children 1 year of age and older, it may be safely given to babies 6 to 12 months of age. Alternatively, babies younger than 1 year of age may be given immune globulin to prevent the infection.

Travellers who have an immune system that doesn't work well may be given immune globulin in addition to vaccine.

For more information on hepatitis A virus and the vaccine that protects against it, see Chapter 10.

Meningococcal vaccine

In Canada, meningococcal group C vaccine is given to all infants routinely, starting at either 12 months or 2 months of age depending on where you live. Travellers may be exposed to other types of meningococci and require the quadrivalent (A-C-Y-W135) meningococcal vaccine. This vaccine is routinely given to teenagers in some parts of Canada and, if needed, can be given to children 2 months of age and older.
- Invasive meningococcal disease occurs worldwide but outbreaks occur frequently in sub-Saharan Africa. Meningococcal vaccine is recommended for travellers to regions experiencing outbreaks of meningococcal disease, especially if they expect to have close contact with the local population. Short-term travellers on business or holiday who will have little contact with local residents are at minimal risk of exposure and immunization may not be required.
- Proof of meningococcal immunization is required for pilgrims travelling to **Saudi Arabia** for Hajj or Umrah.

For more information on meningococcal disease and vaccines, see Chapter 15.

Typhoid fever

Typhoid fever is now rare in Canada and many other countries. Most cases involve people who travel to parts of the world where the disease is still common and where food and water sources may be contaminated. Travellers to Southeast Asia are at highest risk, especially if visiting India, Pakistan and Bangladesh but also Afghanistan, Nepal, the Maldives, Sri Lanka and Bhutan. There is a lower risk for travellers to Africa, the Middle East and parts of South America.

Typhoid fever is caused by bacteria called *Salmonella typhi*. It usually spreads by close contact with an infected person (e.g., if hands are not washed properly after a bowel movement), or by eating food or drinking water contaminated with the bacteria. Bacteria spread from the intestinal tract into the bloodstream.

Typhoid fever is a severe illness. Even with antibiotic treatment, some people die. Symptoms include high fever for a week or more, cough and abdominal pain. Complications occur in about 1% of cases and include perforation of the intestine and intestinal bleeding. Antibiotic treatment is very effective, although many typhoid strains, especially in developing countries, have become resistant to the most commonly used antibiotics.

Precautions are also essential

Since typhoid vaccine is only moderately effective in preventing disease, hygienic precautions such as meticulous handwashing and avoiding possibly-contaminated food or water are very important.

Typhoid fever vaccines

Two different typhoid vaccines are available in Canada.

The **purified polysaccharide vaccine** is made of a complex sugar (polysaccharide) that forms the outer coat of the typhoid bacteria. This polysaccharide is extracted from the bacteria and purified to make the vaccine. Vaccine is injected in a single dose and should be given *at least* 14 days before travel, if possible. Boosters are recommended every 3 years if exposure to typhoid continues.

This vaccine is not recommended for children under 2 years old because it has not been tested in that age group. Pain at the injection site is common but other adverse effects are rare.

The **live attenuated oral vaccine** is made from a weakened strain of typhoid bacteria that multiplies briefly in the intestinal tract, then dies. The vaccine bacteria do not enter the bloodstream and cannot cause typhoid fever. Produced in the form of capsules, this vaccine is swallowed. One capsule is taken every other day, for a total of 4 capsules. All doses should be taken *at least* 7 days before travel, if possible. The live vaccine is recommended only for people 6 years of age and older who can swallow large capsules. A booster is recommended after 7 years if exposure to typhoid continues. Some people experience side effects such as mild nausea and abdominal discomfort.

The live typhoid vaccine is not given to people with acute gastroenteritis or inflammatory bowel disease; nor is it given to people who are immunocompromised. Antibiotics should not be given for 3 days after getting the typhoid vaccine because they will make the vaccine ineffective.

Who should get this vaccine:
- Typhoid vaccine is recommended for **all travellers to Southeast Asia**.
- Typhoid vaccine is not usually required for travel to other areas of the world with higher typhoid rates, such as Africa, parts of the Middle East and South America. It should be considered for **people at high risk of becoming infected** or of **having more severe disease, if infected**, especially if they are likely to be exposed to potentially contaminated food or water. But even for this group, typhoid vaccine may not be needed for short-term holidays in resort hotels.

People at high risk of infection include children, people visiting friends and relatives or staying for a long period of time, and visitors to rural areas. Typhoid fever is more severe in people with reduced stomach acid as a result of disease or medications to suppress acid, people with no spleen or a spleen that isn't working well, and people who are immunocompromised.

Yellow fever

Yellow fever is a severe infection caused by a virus that is found only in some parts of Africa and Central and South America. It is spread by mosquitoes.

Infection with yellow fever virus can cause:
• Hepatitis (acute inflammation of the liver), with symptoms similar to other types of hepatitis (i.e., nausea, abdominal pain, fatigue and jaundice caused by liver malfunction)
• Bleeding (from the nose, mouth, intestinal tract and skin, and into the lungs)
• Death (the death rate is as high as 20%).

Yellow fever vaccine

Yellow fever vaccine is a live attenuated (weakened) virus vaccine. It is grown in chicken eggs. The vaccine is very effective in preventing disease and is recommended for anyone over 9 months of age who travels to a part of the world where yellow fever exists.

The yellow fever vaccine is only given in certain designated travel clinics. Every vaccine recipient receives an International Yellow Fever Vaccine certificate, a document required to enter some countries. The certificate is valid for 10 years, beginning 10 days after immunization. Travellers who need a certificate but cannot be vaccinated because they are younger than 9 months old, have a weakened immune system or some other contraindication to the vaccine (see below) can get an International Certificate of Medical Contraindication to Vaccination. For a list of the Yellow Fever Vaccination Centres, contact your local public health department or refer to the Public Health Agency of Canada's website at: www.phac-aspc.gc.ca/tmp-pmv/yf-fj/index-eng.php

Yellow fever vaccine has few side effects. Reactions to the vaccine are usually mild and brief, and may include headache, muscle aches, and fever. People who have a serious allergy to eggs, chicken or gelatin, and individuals who have had a serious reaction to a previous dose of yellow fever vaccine, should consult with an allergist if yellow fever vaccine is needed.

Serious adverse effects have been reported but are extremely rare. Encephalitis has occurred in children under 6 months old. A few cases of Guillain-Barré syndrome (a type of paralysis) have occurred shortly after vaccination. A more severe disease with fever and a generalized infection may occur in people who are immunocompromised and has occurred (though again, only rarely) in healthy adults over age 60.

Travellers who have a disease or are receiving a treatment that suppresses their immune system should not receive this vaccine. If travel to a yellow fever area is unavoidable, strict precautions against mosquito bites must be taken, such as protective clothing, insect repellants, window screens and bed-nets. For general guidance, see "Insect bite prevention": http://travel.gc.ca/travelling/health-safety/insect-bite. Immunocompromised travellers need to carry a vaccination waiver (International Certificate of Medical Contraindication to Vaccination).

Other people at risk of serious side effects from yellow fever vaccine are:
- **Infants.** The vaccine is recommended for children 9 months of age and older. It is not given to infants under the age of 6 months because of a higher risk of serious side effects. For babies 6 to 8 months old who must travel to an area with yellow fever, the vaccine may be considered.
- **Adults over 60 years old**, although serious effects are rare.
- **Pregnant women.** As with other live vaccines, yellow fever vaccine is not given in pregnancy, unless it's unavoidable.
- **Breastfeeding women.** There have been rare cases of transmission of the vaccine in breast milk.

For these people, the risks of vaccination versus contracting the disease need to be carefully considered. Vaccine should be given only if they are travelling to a high-risk area, travel cannot be postponed, and continual protection against mosquito bites cannot be assured. Otherwise a vaccination waiver should be obtained.

Other vaccines

Other vaccines for travellers may be needed, depending on:
• Destination
• How long a traveller will be away (especially if moving to another country)
• Living conditions (e.g., staying in a hotel or with a local family or visiting relatives and friends; living in a city or a remote village)
• The work or activities a traveller will undertake (e.g., staying at a beach or hiking the forest, exposure to biting insects, animal exposures or hospital work).

Japanese encephalitis

Japanese encephalitis (JE) is a viral infection spread by mosquitoes and found in parts of Asia, especially in the southeast and the western Pacific regions. Although the virus is the leading cause of encephalitis (inflammation of the brain) in Asia, this occurs in only a small proportion of cases. Most people get a flu-like illness with fever and muscle aches. Symptoms of encephalitis include fever, severe headache, vomiting, convulsions and impaired consciousness.

Japanese encephalitis vaccine is a purified, inactivated vaccine prepared in cell cultures. It is safe and very effective in preventing disease. Given by injection, 2 doses are required, 28 days apart, with vaccination completed 10 days before travel. Local injection site reactions are common. General reactions such as headache, muscle aches and fever are less common.

The risk for acquiring JE is low for most travellers, particularly for short-term visitors to major urban areas. The mosquito that carries JE is found mainly in rural areas.

JE vaccine is only recommended for travellers to countries where the virus is found, who will be there during the transmission season (summer and fall in temperate areas and year-round in tropical areas) and who will have a high risk of exposure. These include:

- Travellers who will spend more than 30 days in rural areas or in urban areas known to have JE, long-term travellers, and people moving to live in an affected country who may be making repeated short trips to rural areas.
- Travellers who will spend less than 30 days in areas with JE, if they expect to spend a lot of time outdoors or if indoor mosquito control is poor, especially during the evenings and at night.

In Canada, JE vaccine is licensed only for adults, but a similar vaccine is licensed for children in other parts of the world. For children at risk, such as when protection from mosquitoes cannot be assured, the adult vaccine may be used. The paediatric vaccine may also be obtained at the travel destination, if time permits.

Tick-borne encephalitis

Tick-borne encephalitis (TBE) is a viral disease affecting the brain. It is spread by biting ticks found in various parts of Europe, Russia and the Far East. These ticks are found near the edges of forests and in wooded areas, parks, meadows and grasslands. Ticks are active from March to November in central Europe. Activities like hiking, bicycling or camping outdoors increase the likelihood of contact with ticks, and taking precautions against tick bites (e.g., wearing protective clothing and using insect repellants) is recommended. For general guidance, see "Insect bite prevention": http://travel.gc.ca/travelling/health-safety/insect-bite

Tick-borne encephalitis (TBE) vaccine is available in Canada and may be given to travellers to countries where TBE exists if they are at risk of tick bites, which depends on the season of travel and activities planned. The vaccine is safe and effective.

TBE vaccine is an inactivated virus vaccine made in chick cell cultures. It is given by injection in 2 doses at least 14 days apart, with a third dose at 3 to 15 months if the person is still in an area where TBE occurs. Local injection site reactions are common, and fever is also common in young children. Serious adverse effects are very rare.

The vaccine is licensed in Canada only for people 16 years of age and older. A paediatric form of the same vaccine is available in Europe. For children needing vaccination, the European paediatric vaccine may be obtained through Health Canada's Special Access Program, or a half-dose of the adult vaccine may be used. The vaccine may also be obtained at the travel destination, if time permits.

Travellers' diarrhea and cholera

A single vaccine available in Canada protects against both travellers' diarrhea and cholera.

Travellers' diarrhea: Up to 50% of travellers from developed countries who visit developing countries get travellers' diarrhea. The highest rates are seen in travellers to Latin America, Africa and India, with lower rates in travellers to China, Russia, the Middle East and Southeast Asia. A bacteria, enterotoxigenic *Escherichia coli* (ETEC), is the most common cause of travellers' diarrhea, accounting for 25% to 50% of cases. Most episodes of travellers' diarrhea are mild and get better without treatment. Infection spreads through contaminated food and water.

Preventing travellers' diarrhea depends more on attention to safe food, clean water and careful hand hygiene than on immunization. The vaccine is of limited benefit because it protects against ETEC only. It provides short-term protection, and boosters are needed every 3 months. Antibiotics are sometimes used to prevent travellers' diarrhea.

Vaccine is recommended only for high-risk travellers who may become severely ill if they get ETEC. Especially vulnerable are people who are immunocompromised, individuals with chronic renal failure, congestive heart failure, insulin-dependent diabetes, or inflammatory bowel disease, and those taking medications that suppress stomach acid.

Cholera: Cholera causes severe watery diarrhea. If left untreated, fluid loss can lead to rapid dehydration and life-threatening shock. Cholera is caused by *Vibrio cholerae* bacteria, and spreads through contaminated water or food. It is found in several countries but the risk of spread is highest in disaster situations, when water and sanitation systems are disrupted or populations are displaced or living in overcrowded camps.

Most travellers to countries affected by cholera are unlikely to get the infection. Preventing cholera depends more on access to safe food and water and careful hand hygiene than on immunization. At higher risk are people who ingest contaminated water or food (especially undercooked or raw shellfish or fish) and those visiting or working in areas of cholera outbreaks with limited access to safe water and food.

The vaccine may benefit travellers who are at significant risk of exposure (such as humanitarian workers or health professionals going to work in a country with a cholera outbreak) or who are immunocompromised, and therefore at risk of severe illness if they become infected.

Cholera and travellers' diarrhea vaccine is an inactivated, oral vaccine. It is provided as a liquid that must be mixed with a sodium bicarbonate buffer (also provided) and drunk. The vaccine is not recommended for children under 2 years old because it has not been studied in this age group. The most common adverse events connected with this vaccine are stomach pain, diarrhea, nausea and vomiting. These symptoms are probably caused by the bicarbonate buffer, not the vaccine.

For travellers' diarrhea, 2 doses are needed, 1 to 6 weeks apart. For cholera, children 2 to 5 years of age need 3 doses, 1 to 6 weeks apart, and people 6 years of age and older need 2 doses, 1 to 6 weeks apart. Doses should be completed *at least* a week before travelling. Protection against ETEC lasts 3 months, while cholera protection lasts for 6 months in children 2 to 5 years of age, and for 2 years in people 6 years of age and older.

Rabies

People get rabies from being bitten by an infected dog, other pet or wild animal. Rabies is a virus that attacks the brain and infection is usually fatal. Fortunately, vaccine and immune globulin given soon after the animal bite prevent disease.

Rabies is more common in many developing countries than in Canada, and effective vaccines for treatment if a bite occurs are not always available in those countries. Travellers to areas where rabies is common and adequate treatment for animal bites may be less available or reliable should consider being immunized against rabies, especially if they plan an extended stay. Their destination, purpose and length of stay, lifestyle, planned activities and the likelihood of animal exposure should all be considered. Children are at higher risk of bites, especially if they are too young to understand the need to avoid animals or to report an animal bite.

Rabies vaccine is an inactivated virus vaccine made in cell culture. It can be given by injection to children and adults of any age. If given before travelling, 3 doses are needed, the second at 7 days and the third 21 to 28 days after the first. If given after a bite, 4 doses are needed at more frequent intervals, and rabies immune globulin is also given.

Tuberculosis

Bacille Calmette-Guérin (BCG) vaccine is needed only rarely, but may be considered for some travellers planning an extended stay in areas or countries with high rates of tuberculosis, where contact with the disease is likely, and other protective measures are not available. Consultation with a travel medicine specialist is recommended. The vaccine is a live bacteria vaccine and can be given to people of any age, including newborns. As for other live vaccines, BCG should not be given to people who are immunocompromised.

Index

A page number *in italics* indicates that the information is in a table or figure on that page.

HPV *see* human papillomavirus (HPV)
HSCT (hematopoietic stem cell transplantation), 34
human papillomavirus (HPV) infection
    cause, 187–88
    complications/seriousness, 6, 185
    diagnosis, 190
    history, 186–87
    risk–benefit comparison with vaccine, 107, *109*
    spread, 188
    symptoms, 189–90
    treatment, 190
human papillomavirus (HPV) vaccine
    additives/other substances, 54, 56
    effectiveness, 193–94
    history, 187
    how given, 191
    how it is maade, 191
    risk–benefit comparison with disease, 107, *109*
    side effects, 193
    types and forms, 190, 191
    vaccination schedule, 18, 19, 191–92
hypotensive-hyporesponsive events, 91, 269

– I –
illness *see* diseases
immigrants
    hepatitis A vaccination, *164*
    hepatitis B vaccination, *179*
    information resource, 343
    vaccine "catch-up" doses, 13
immune globulin
    for chickenpox, 124–25
    for children with congenital immunodeficiency, 32
    for hepatitis A, 165–66
    for hepatitis B, 179–80, *181*
    for measles, 225–26
    for tetanus, 334, 336
    for use after exposures, 37
    vaccine interactions, 127, 130, 229, 256, 327
immune memory *see* immunity
immune system
    purpose, 41
    and quantity of vaccines, 47
    response to germs, 42–43
immunity
    duration, 45–46
    infection-specific, *43*
    long-term, 43
    with natural infection, 43–45
    passive, 47–49
    short-term, 42
    with vaccines, 44–45
immunization *see* vaccination
Immunization Action Coalition (U.S.), 345–46
Immunization Safety Review Committee (U.S.), 74–75
Immunize Canada, 341, 344
immunocompromising conditions
    and chickenpox, 121, 126–27
    and Hib disease, *154*
    and influenza vaccine, 211
    and measles vaccine, 227, 228
    and mumps vaccine, 255
    and pneumococcal disease, *290*
    and rotavirus vaccine, 312–13
    and rubella vaccine, 326
    and shingles vaccine, 130
    and travel, 39
    and vaccine needs, 31–32, 96
immunosuppressive therapy
    and vaccine cautions, 28–29
    and vaccine needs, 36
IMPACT (Canadian Immunization Monitoring Program, ACTive), 72–73, 76
inactivated polio vaccine (IPV) *see* polio vaccine
India
    travellers' diarrhea, 357
    typhoid fever, 351

Indonesia, polio, 295
Infanrix, 56
infantile spasms, *not* caused by pertussis vaccine, 101, *270*, 271
infants
    antibodies from mother, 48, 230, 294
    premature, *16*, *48*
    reducing vaccination pain, 61–64
    routine vaccines, 14–15
infections
    as beneficial, 10
    body's response to, 42–43, 44
    how they start, 42
    natural, 44–45, *46*
    not caused by vaccines, 228
    serious complications and death from, 5–7
inflammatory bowel disease, 28
inflammatory diseases, 28–29, *30*
influenza
    A and B virus strains, 198
    avian, 199–200
    and babies, 15
    cause, 200
    complications/seriousness, 6, 195, 201–2
    diagnosis, 202
    history, 196–98
    pandemics, 195–97, 199
    risk–benefit comparison with vaccine, *109*
    spread, 200–201
    symptoms, 201
    treatment, 203
influenza vaccine
    additives/other substances, 53, 54, 55–56
    cost, *198*
    effectiveness, 212–13
    history, 197–98
    how given, 207
    how it is made, 205–6
    for infants, 15
    for older adults, 20
    for people with chronic conditions, *24*, 25, 27–29, *30*
    for people with immunocompromising conditions, 33–36
    for pregnant women, 20
    risk–benefit comparison with disease, *109*
    side effects, 209–10
    types and forms, 204, 206–7
    vaccination schedule, 17, 18, 209
    when to delay/avoid, 93, 210–12
    who should get it, 207–8, *208*
information *see* resources
Institute of Medicine (U.S.), 346
Internet
    evaluating sites, 340–42
    misinformation, 2, 11, 339, 341–42
    reliable information, 2, 57, 84, 343–47
intussusception, 97, 312, 313
invasive meningococcal disease *see* meningococcal disease
itchiness at injection site, 91

– J –
Japan
    acellular vaccines, 266
    autism study, 99
    chickenpox vaccine, 122
    pertussis and vaccine, 273–74, *273*, 275
    rubella vaccine, 323
Japanese encephalitis, 39, 355
Japanese encephalitis vaccine, 39, 355–56
jaundice
    defined, 158
    with hepatitis A, 158, 161
    with hepatitis B, 175
joint infection
    from Hib, 149, 150
    from pneumococcal infection, 283
joint pain, 91, 227